MIDWIFERY PRACTICE:

Core Topics 3

Edited by

Jo Alexander, Carolyn Roth

© Series Selection: Jo Alexander, Valerie Levy & Sarah Roch 1990, 1993, 1995, 1996; Jo Alexander, Carolyn Roth & Valerie Levy 1997, 2000

© This volume: Foreword, Cathy Warwick; Reflections on midwifery care and the postnatal period, Tricia Anderson and Jane Podkolinski; The need to talk after birth: evaluating new services, Sally Marchant and Jo Garcia; Perinatal grief: understanding the bereaved and their carers, Rosemary Mander; From pregnancy to lactation: changing relations between mother and baby – a biological perspective, Mary McNabb and Suzanne Colson; Breastfeeding update, Sally Inch; Sexual health in the postnatal period, Jill Stewart-Moore; Domestic violence and pregnancy: a midwifery issue, Chris Bewley and Andy Gibbs; Empowerment – a gift bestowed or withheld?, Gillian Fletcher and Elisabeth Buggins; Organisation of postnatal care and related issues, Debra Bick, 2000

First published 2000 by
MACMILLAN PRESS LTD
Houndmills, Basingstoke, Hampshire RG21 6XS
and London
Companies and representatives
throughout the world

ISBN 0–333–76433–1 paperback

A catalogue record for this book is available
from the British Library.

This book is printed on paper suitable for recycling and
made from fully managed and sustained forest sources.

10 9   8   7   6   5   4   3   2   1
09 08 07 06 05 04 03 02 01 00

Editing and origination by
Aardvark Editorial, Mendham, Suffolk

Printed and bound in Great Britain by
Creative Print & Design (Wales), Ebbw Vale

Contents

Other volumes in the Midwifery Practice series

■ **Midwifery practice: Core topics 1**   ISBN 0–333–66320–9

Rosemary Currell: The organisation of maternity care
Greta Curtis: Preconception care
Jennifer Wilson: Antenatal risk assessment
Colin Rees: Antenatal education, health promotion and the midwife
Elsa Montgomery: Fetal wellbeing: the intrauterine environment and ensuing legal and clinical issues
Jane Denton: Pregnancy after treatment for infertility
Helen R. Minns: Women with learning disabilities: the midwife's role
Tansy M. Cheston: Pre-eclampsia
Kathleen King: Marketing midwifery services

■ **Midwifery practice: Core topics 2**   ISBN 0–333–69627–1

Rona Campbell: Place of birth reconsidered
Carole Yearley: Motherhood as a rite of passage: an anthropological perspective
Chris Bewley and Cliff Roberts: Injectable methods of pain relief in labour
Sue McDonald: Active management of labour
Maxine Wallis-Redworth: Emergencies during labour: umbilical cord prolapse and inversion of the uterus
Tansy M. Cheston: Diabetes mellitus in pregnancy
Rona McCandlish: Care during the second stage of labour
Juliet Wood and Jane Rogers: The third stage of labour
Carol Bates: Care in normal labour: a feminist perspective

■ **Aspects of midwifery practice**   ISBN 0–333–61956–0

Sally Spedding, Joan Wilson, Sarah Wright and Alan Jackson: Nutrition for pregnancy and lactation
Rosaline Steele: Midwifery care in the first stage of labour
Elaine Carty: Disability, pregnancy and parenting
Terri Coates: Shoulder dystocia
Catherine Siney: Drug addicted mothers
Carolyn Roth: HIV and pregnancy
Jennifer Sleep: Postnatal perineal care revisited
Susan L. Smith: Neonatal hypoglycaemia
Sally Marchant and Jo Garcia: Routine clinical care in the immediate postnatal period

Contributors to this volume

Tricia Anderson BA (Hons), MSc, RM
Lecturer in Midwifery/Independent Midwife, Institute of Health and Community Studies, Bournemouth University
Tricia Anderson trained as a midwife in Dorset, where she worked in both hospital and community settings before commencing independent practice in 1997. She was formerly Editor of the *MIDIRS Midwifery Digest* and Co-editor of the *Informed Choice Initiative*. She is now Associate Editor of *Practising Midwife* and part-time lecturer in midwifery studies.

Chris Bewley MSc, BEd, RN, RM, ADM
Senior Lecturer in Midwifery, Middlesex University
Chris Bewley has 10 years' experience of writing and speaking on the subject of domestic violence and pregnancy. She has also written about interpersonal and educational issues relating to midwifery and co-contributed a chapter on 'Injectable methods of pain relief' to the previous volume in this series.

Debra Bick BA, MMedSci, RGN, RM
Research Fellow in Midwifery, University of Birmingham
Debra Bick's main research interests concern aspects of maternal health after childbirth. She is currently involved with two large randomised controlled trials, the results of which will inform evidence-based care for women during labour and the puerperium.

Elisabeth Buggins MHSM, DipHSM
Chairman Walsall Community Health NHS Trust
Elisabeth Buggins has a wide experience of involvement with both the NHS and the voluntary sector. Now Chairman of Walsall Community Health NHS Trust, and of Wolverhampton MSLC, she aims to build strong, multi-disciplinary, multiagency teams that work constructively to effect change.

Suzanne Colson RGN RM BA Licence ès Lettres (France)
Rosie Maternity Hospital, Cambridge
Suzanne Colson is clinical facilitator for research and development in transitional care. For her MSc thesis, she is examining aspects of suckling ketosis. She has worked as baby feeding advisor at Pithiviers Hospital, France and the Royal Free Hospital, London where she was seconded to UCH to complete breastfeeding research concerning metabolic adaptation in the preterm infant.

Gillian Fletcher MCSP, NCT Antenatal Tutor
Freelance Trainer
Gillian Fletcher has been involved in antenatal and postnatal work for 27 years and was responsible for setting up the NCT teacher training programme in Europe. With a physiotherapist colleague, she developed the NCT postnatal exercise training programme. Gillian is author of *Get Into Shape After Childbirth*, and is currently working on a user involvement project with the College of Health.

Jo Garcia BA, MSc
Social Scientist, National Perinatal Epidemiology Unit, Oxford
Jo Garcia is currently Director of the Midwifery Research Programme at the NPEU. She has written widely and has contributed, with Sally Marchant, to a previous volume in the series.

Andy Gibbs
Head of Department of Child Health, Mental Health and Learning Disabilities, Napier University, Edinburgh
Andy Gibbs is also Research Fellow for the National Board for Nursing, Midwifery and Health Visiting for Scotland and is currently researching midwives' experiences of interventions with regard to domestic abuse.

Sally Inch RM, RN
Breastfeeding Advisor and Baby Friendly Co-ordinator for the Women's Centre, John Radcliffe Hospital, Oxford
As well as her two books on aspects of birth, *Birthrights* and *Approaching Birth*, Sally Inch has written widely on the subject of breastfeeding, co-authoring, editing and contributing to numerous books, papers, articles and videos. Since May 1998, she has worked with Chloe Fisher in the Oxford Breastfeeding Clinic.

Mary McNabb MSc, BA, RN, RM, ADM, PGCEA
Senior Lecturer, South Bank University
Mary McNabb has a longstanding interest in reproductive biology and social ecology. She has written the biology chapters for the current edition of *Mayes' Midwifery* and is currently working on a chapter on embryo formation and fetal development, for a forthcoming physiologically based textbook on child health.

Rosemary Mander MSc, PhD, RGN, SCM, MTD
Reader, Department of Nursing Studies, University of Edinburgh
Rosemary Mander is involved with teaching at postgraduate level, as well as undertaking research. She has an honorary appointment that facilitates her practice as a midwife at a local maternity unit. Her activities in the university and in the maternity unit both serve to inform her writing on midwifery-related topics.

Sally Marchant RN, RM, ADM, Diploma in Research Methods
Research Midwife, National Perinatal Epidemiology Unit, Oxford
Sally Marchant's main interest is in women's health following childbirth, particularly in the ways in which midwifery care can help to reduce women's morbidity, both physical and psychological, during the postnatal period.

Jane Podkolinski BA (Econ), MSc, SRN, SCM, DPSM
Practising Midwife
Jane Podkolinski has a first degree in economics. She then began to train as an accountant, but in 1975 changed direction to pursue a career in nursing. She qualified as a midwife in 1979 and has been working since then in all aspects of clinical midwifery in both hospital and community settings.

Jill Stewart-Moore RN, RM, MTD, MSc
Chair of the Management Committee of Belfast Brook Advisory Centre
Jill Stewart-Moore has experience of family planning, nursing and midwifery lecturing in South London and now Belfast.

Foreword

As a midwife, the provision of postnatal care has always fascinated me. Many commonly held beliefs about this important period in women's lives have never quite made sense. Could it really be unsafe for a mother to cuddle her baby in bed with her? Were small four-bedded bays automatically a superior hospital design in which to care for women? Why was it considered that women having their first baby would fare better staying in hospital longer than women having their second or third baby? The complete opposite of what was common practice often seemed far more logical. As a community midwife, I solemnly carried out the ritual physical examination of mother and baby but, at an early stage in my career, I doubted that it was the examinations in themselves that were of most importance. Was it not something about the interaction they necessitated between the mother and the midwife?

Now, as a midwifery manager, I can see clearly that one of our greatest challenges as a profession is to try to understand what it is about the postnatal period that matters to women and how the care we give can best enable women to fulfil their role as mothers. As Tricia Anderson and Jane Podkolinski point out in the book's introductory chapter, postnatal care throughout the country is poorly evaluated. Surveys of user opinion suggest that midwives struggle to perform a set of rituals of unproven value while failing to provide the support women really want or need. Community midwives have adopted patterns of selective visiting with the overt aim of tailoring care more specifically to the needs of women, but it is hard not to be cynical and imagine that the tailoring has something to do with the workload and pressures experienced by the midwives.

It would be wrong to be too negative, and that is quite rightly not the tone of the book. Care provision has changed and, all over the country, patterns of care based on available evidence are developing. Furthermore, the authors of this book, in their presentation of the theoretical basis for care and of the evidence, frequently support the fact that certain current practices are both justifiable and useful. This will very importantly build the confidence of practitioners. I do quite deliberately use the term 'practitioners'. The book is not directed at one professional group. In fact, many authors specifically mention the need for a multidisciplinary approach, and midwives, GPs, health visitors, paediatricians and obstetricians could all benefit from the insights and ideas contained in the various chapters.

I hope that the greatest contribution of this book will be to help professionals to look at postnatal care differently and to consider how their practice might alter. The book specifically attempts to promote change through its style of concluding each chapter with a section encouraging professionals to consider their own practice or their own service in the light of what they have read. This is a very welcome step. Theories and ideas are all very well, but it is widely understood that they do not in themselves ensure that care improves.

Important themes recur throughout the book. Two of these are the need to treat women as individuals and the need to ask the users of the services what matters to them. It may be surprising that such issues still need emphasis, but, in my experience, the focus on providing individualised and women-centred care has concentrated on the antenatal and labour periods. Furthermore, this is about getting things right not just for individual women but for all women – it is about changing policy and the content of care, not just about doing the same things differently.

Of course, radical change is unsettling. If the old rituals of postnatal care are invalid, what do professionals do? The beauty of the book is that it offers positive ways forward. Women need to talk (Chapter 2); domestic violence presents a major challenge (Chapter 7); promoting women's sexual health can avoid much unhappiness and morbidity (Chapter 6). Professionals should adopt a much broader perspective than in the past.

Research is emphasised throughout the book. The various authors present research evidence to counteract widely held beliefs and myths and to suggest alternative ways in which professionals might practise. There is, however, a real danger in slipping from one set of discredited practices into a new set of unproven rituals. Very importantly, authors, particularly Sally Marchant and Jo Garcia, emphasise the need to evaluate new practices. It is encouraging, particularly in Debra Bick's chapter, to see that large-scale research projects into the organisation of postnatal care have recently been funded.

Although the issue of ethics is not specifically addressed, it is interesting to note how frequently the question emerges of whether or not care is ethical. In her chapter on breastfeeding, Sally Inch argues that it would be both patronising and dishonest to withhold the facts about the benefits of breastfeeding to protect the woman from 'feeling guilty'. Chris Bewley raises a rather different point when, in discussing the importance of screening for domestic violence, she points out that it 'would be unethical to encourage disclosure in the absence of a sound supportive infrastructure and system for referral'. It is issues like these that highlight for me that this is an important book which must be read by policy-makers as well as practitioners if we are to achieve optimum care.

It is important to point out, however, that even where a practice is considered 'right', the authors do not imply that this justifies its automatic imposition on women. Sally Inch goes on to say that 'having ascertained that the mother has made an informed choice, health professionals have a duty to support the mother in her choice and assist her to bottle feed safely'. It is this emphasis on getting care right for individuals that emerges again and again.

Perhaps what strikes me most in reading this book is that providing postnatal care is not straightforward. The story that illustrates this most profoundly is the tale of how human milk banks were closed in the late 1980s because of a fear of HIV transmission. This was despite evidence of the effectiveness of pasteurisation in destroying the virus and just before there was overwhelming evidence that there was an increased risk of necrotising enterocolitis in preterm infants who were excessively formula fed. It is easy to criticise professionals for getting it wrong, but perhaps what is most surprising is how often they manage to negotiate all the hurdles and give a good service. It is apt that a final theme of this book, which is particularly emphasised in Gillian Fletcher and Elisabeth Buggins' chapter on empowerment, is that if professionals are to help mothers, they themselves will need support and appropriate education.

This is a book in which the authors examine the art and science of postnatal care. It will, I hope, make a valuable contribution as we continuously strive to provide a service of excellence. It is, I contend, impossible to read this book and not reflect on how one's current practice might change for the better.

Cathy Warwick
KINGS NHS TRUST

Preface

The planning of this book, the eighth volume in the Midwifery Practice series, coincided with the publication of the Audit Commission report *First class delivery* (1997) which revealed that women are more critical about hospital postnatal services than about any other aspect of their maternity care. The report highlighted the considerable variation that exists in the way in which postnatal care is organised and the level to which it is resourced; it stressed the need for clear objectives, quality standards and genuine partnership with women.

The issues raised in the report have important implications for midwives as the reappraisal of the needs of women, babies and families in the postnatal period demands a critical assessment of the knowledge, skills and perspectives of midwives giving postnatal care. In our opinion, postnatal care has a vital role to play in promoting health in its broadest sense, and we hope that what follows will make a contribution to the important debate on what that care should include.

Throughout this series, our intention as editors has been to encourage midwives' access to sound, well-referenced material that addresses issues arising within their clinical practice. The series has developed alongside the increasing access to and use by midwives of tools such as the Cochrane Library and the MIRIAD Midwifery Research Database, as well as a proliferation of critical discussion on midwifery knowledge and practice, reflected in the growing number of research-based midwifery journals. We believe this series provides an additional resource for the benefit both of those with a limited opportunity for inquiry and those wishing to investigate topics further.

We are grateful for the work of all our contributors. They have critically appraised a wide range of literature and evidence of relevance to midwifery practice. The collection will, we hope, stimulate readers' consideration of a range of research approaches and sources of knowledge that can enhance their understanding of midwifery practice and the challenges it presents. We believe that the current edition continues our objective to strengthen the dynamic links between education, practice and research.

Finally we would like to thank our publishers, especially our outstanding publishers' editor, Richenda Milton-Thompson, and Carrie Walker our copy-editor.

Jo Alexander, Carolyn Roth, Val Levy

■ Common structure of the chapters

In fulfilment of the aims of the series, each chapter follows a common structure:

1. The introduction offers a digest of the contents;

2. 'It is assumed that you are already aware of the following...' establishes the prerequisite knowledge and experience assumed of the reader;

3. The main body of the chapter then reviews and analyses the most appropriate and important research literature currently available;

4. The 'Recommendations for clinical practice' offer suggestions for sound clinical practice, based on the author's interpretation of the literature;

5. The 'Practice check' enables professionals to examine their own practice and the principles and policies influencing their work;

6. Bibliographic sources are covered under 'References' and 'Suggested further reading'.

■ Reference

Audit Commission (1997) First class delivery: improving maternity services in England and Wales. Audit Commission, London

■ Suggested further reading on research

Couchman W, Dawson J (1995) Nursing and Healthcare Research, 2nd edn. Scutari Press, London.
Distance Learning Centre modules (1987–95) Research Awareness: A Programme for Nurses, Midwives and Health Visitors, Units 1–11. South Bank University, London.
Hicks C (1990) Research and Statistics: A Practical Introduction for Nurses. Prentice Hall, Hemel Hempstead.
Parahoo K (1997) Nursing Research: Principles, Process, Issues. Macmillan, Basingstoke.
Polit DF, Hungler BP (1995) Nursing Research: Principles and Methods, 5th edn. JB Lippincott, Philadelphia.
Robson C (1993) Real World Research: A Resource For Social Scientists and Practitioner-researchers. Blackwell, Oxford.

Acknowledgements

Every effort has been made to trace all copyright holders, but if any have been inadvertently overlooked, the publishers will be pleased to make the necessary arrangements at the first opportunity.

Chapter 1

Reflections on midwifery care and the postnatal period

Tricia Anderson and Jane Podkolinski

■ Introduction

What are we trying to achieve by the provision of midwifery postnatal care? One of the recommendations in the Audit Commission's recent review of the maternity services is that 'clinicians and managers in trusts should clarify the objectives and set standards for postnatal care in hospital and at home' (Audit Commission 1997: 65).

> There is... some uncertainty about what postnatal care is aiming to achieve – whether it is solely to prevent and treat immediate health problems in mother and baby or whether it is aiming to enhance the overall experience, giving mothers time to recover and get to know their babies, possibly avoiding other problems later on.
> (Audit Commission 1997: 52)

Contemporary midwifery textbooks describe theoretical aims for postnatal care and the role of the midwife during the postnatal period as promoting the physical well-being of women and their babies; meeting their psychological and emotional needs; giving support that includes health education about caring for the baby; helping to establish infant feeding; and facilitating a successful transition to parenthood (Ball 1993; Silverton 1993; Parr *et al* 1997; Sweet 1997).

Why, then, does postnatal practice continue to focus on performing routine physical observations to screen for maternal and neonatal morbidity? The majority of midwives still check a woman's breasts and nipples, rate of uterine involution, lochia, perineum, legs and urinary function on a daily basis (Marchant 1995). Midwives' postnatal records of their care are testimony to this. Much of this routinised care has not changed for 70 years or more and is based on the historical premise that women are at risk of developing puerperal fever, a condition no longer highly relevant in Western culture as a result of the introduction of anti-

1

biotics (Garcia & Marchant 1996), better living conditions and better diet (Oakley 1979). Contemporary postnatal care is also based on a spurious intent to monitor a woman's body as it 'returns to normal' by the end of the postnatal period (currently defined as 6 weeks after the birth). Maclean (1994) describes how childbirth should leave a woman at least as healthy as she was before pregnancy, and Sweet (1997: 475) claims that 'it takes between 6 and 12 weeks for most women to return to their normal emotional state'. But where is the evidence to support these statements? And what constitutes 'normal'?

Women's lives and bodies are fundamentally changed, both physically and psychologically, by the process of parturition and motherhood, and there is a growing body of evidence that professionals may not be meeting women's needs for care at this time. In one large study, 67 per cent of women had at least one health problem after childbirth lasting for a minimum of 6 weeks and often much longer, and 35 per cent of women experienced new health problems that they had not had prior to giving birth and that lasted for over a year after childbirth (MacArthur *et al* 1991). Another study found more than three-quarters (76 per cent) of women reporting symptoms that persisted beyond 8 weeks after birth (Glazener *et al* 1993a, 1993b). Women talk of persistent backache, headaches, urinary incontinence, perineal pain, sexual difficulties, depression and overwhelming tiredness. Many women struggle on in silence for years with chronic health problems that originated from their childbirth experience, yet never seek help (MacArthur *et al* 1991; Dewan *et al* 1993; Bick & MacArthur 1995).

The widespread incidence of these perinatal symptoms suggests that they are not abnormal findings; on the contrary, if we define normal as meaning 'commonly occurring', they are a normal part of early mother-hood. Neither is the morbidity simply related to complicated deliveries: 17 per cent of women who had an intact perineum at delivery were experiencing painful sexual intercourse a year after delivery (Johanson *et al* 1993). Furthermore, it appears that the postnatal care we currently provide does little, if anything, to diagnose, treat or cure the health problems associated with childbirth.

Finally, women are not happy with the postnatal care they receive: 'Women make more negative comments about postnatal hospital services than any other aspects of their maternity care' (Audit Commission 1997: 50). In the Audit Commission report, over a quarter of women complained of conflicting advice on breastfeeding, 38 per cent felt that they had no say in when they went home from hospital, 40 per cent saw three or more different midwives for their postnatal visits, hospital facilities were described as poor, and over 20 per cent of women felt that the frequency of postnatal visits was inappropriate for them (Audit Commission 1997). Similarly, Glazener *et al* (1993) found that by 8 weeks after the birth, only just over half of women thought the postnatal care was very good.

This chapter aims to explore the reasons why postnatal care fails for so many women, suggesting other factors that need to be taken into consideration when providing care for women after childbirth.

■ It is assumed that you are already aware of the following:

- The physiological and psychological changes that occur in the puerperium;
- The current NHS provision of postnatal care in the UK;
- The UKCC Midwives' Rules and Code of Practice relating to the provision of postnatal care;
- The cultural context of the women you look after.

■ Postnatal care and the medical model

Much of current midwifery knowledge used to underpin practice has been dictated by the growing dominance of the obstetric profession, whose own knowledge base is founded on a 'medical model'. This dominance has escalated over the past 40 years with the development of high technology such as ultrasound scans and fetal monitors to view the fetus (Oakley 1993). To accommodate these developments, the place of delivery has moved from home to hospital. Thereby, the medical 'experts', who claim special status and financial reward because of their expertise in using the new technologies associated with birth, have displaced female friends and family, who traditionally supported women through childbirth (Oakley 1979; Jordan 1987).

The medical model derives from a 17th century world view articulated by Descartes of a mechanistic universe following predictable, repeatable laws that could be discovered by science and controlled by technology. At the heart of the medical model is the notion of 'the body as machine', a machine that can be measured and tested, dissected and analysed, and ultimately repaired. This model views the concept of ill health as a mechanical malfunction on a physiological, pathological level. However, the prototype that the medical model takes as its standard is the male body (Martin 1989). By deviating from the male standard, the female body is 'regarded as inherently abnormal, defective, dangerously unpredictable and under the influence of nature, and in need of constant manipulation by men' (Helman 1994: 147). The medical view sees pregnancy as a wayward, abhorrent and potentially dangerous deviant condition, to be monitored, controlled and corrected until the body is returned to its 'normal' state. Although the postnatal period attracts less attention from obstetricians, the business of birth having been completed, the philosophy espoused by the medical model is still clearly apparent in the symptom checklists used to structure most postnatal care in the UK.

The medical model has been challenged as being an inappropriate metaphor for childbirth, which is a normal life event (Davis-Floyd 1992). By viewing pregnancy and parturition as an aberration from 'normality', the medical model denies the reality of women's lives. It misleads women with regard to the reality of the state of motherhood by implying that they will 'get back to normal' after a certain period of time. Having invested women with the 'sick role' during pregnancy and birth, the medical model pronounces women 'cured' after they have given birth: they are no longer 'sick' and are encouraged to resume normal life as quickly as possible. No wonder women feel unprepared. The state of motherhood and the behaviour of young babies seem far away from the world of controllable, predictable, scientific laws. Efforts to 'get back to normal' may serve only to reinforce the inadequacy and low self-esteem felt by many women as they struggle to adapt their lives to new motherhood (Price 1988).

■ The cultural context of birth

Birth is a biological process, and it is therefore important for midwives to have a knowledge of medicine and physiology to be able to keep women and their babies safe (Kirkham 1996). But how birth is celebrated and new mothers cared for are culturally determined.

Jordan (1993), examining childbirth from an anthropological perspective, proposes that the cultural and social context of birth is as important to a woman's experience of birth and her well-being as is her physical care. Women experience birth within a cultural context that includes social rules and rituals conveying beliefs and values important to the society in which they live. Applying Jordan's insights about women's experience of childbirth suggests that the origin of some of the common problems of the postnatal period should be sought not in physical adaptations after birth but in social ones. In particular, such problems may reflect social expectations that ignore the impact – social, emotional and physical – of childbirth on a woman. Therefore to concentrate on any possible physical causes for women's 'ill-health' postnatally and to treat these with medical solutions may be to ignore other relevant factors that have a bearing on women's well-being.

Thus, many so-called 'problems' can be shown to be culturally constructed. The Western cultural image of normal family life includes women resuming a full sexual relationship with their partner within weeks of giving birth (Robinson 1998). The 6-week check was instigated to assess whether a woman was fit to resume her 'normal' life, which included marital relations (Limerick 1939), yet nearly 50 per cent of women experience difficulties relating to intercourse in the year after childbirth (Glazener 1997). These so-called 'problems' are tiredness, soreness and lack of interest.

By way of contrast, in many traditional African cultures, a woman, who will be breastfeeding, is not expected to resume sexual relations with her husband for anything up to 2 years following the birth. Lefeber and Voorhoeve (1998: 80), on the basis of their anthropological research over many years, write 'it should be realised that abstinence during at least the first year after childbirth is the general custom in indigenous communities'. So whose 'problem' is this 'lack of interest'? From where have women learnt that they should be resuming intercourse with their partners within a matter of weeks of giving birth?

A study of Asian women's experiences of postnatal care in East London (Woollett & Dosanjh-Matwala 1990) also demonstrates how clearly the postnatal period is culturally defined. Asian women reported that their central concern is their need for rest and recovery after childbirth. They expect to forgo their 'normal' duties and be taken care of, receiving substantial family support for several weeks while they recuperate. It is worth noting that it is only in the past 30 years that women in the UK have been expected to manage with minimal domestic support in the postnatal period. As recently as the late 1960s, childbearing women were provided with a home help for the first week after the birth if they did not have help, usually from their own mother (Thomson 1996). Yet in the 1990s, women receive little support and are often expected to be back at work within 3 months or less of giving birth.

■ The medicalisation of sadness

The way in which the distress experienced by women during the postnatal period is understood provides a useful example of how women's feelings about their change in circumstances are interpreted differently depending upon the perspective that is adopted.

Two out of three women (63 per cent) report feeling depressed during the first 9 months following childbirth (McIntosh 1993). This experience of misery (Oakley 1981) is in stark contrast with the notion of the contented mother so widely projected in the popular press and advertising media. Implicit in the medical approach to 'correct' this malfunction is the assumption that the fault lies in the woman: 'Babies should bring happiness but if they do not something is wrong' (Dalton 1989: 154). Female hormones provide a convenient scientific scapegoat, having deviated from their normal, non-pregnant 'setting'. Alternatively, the woman herself is deemed to be at fault for failing to get back to normal, which includes 'getting and recovering from the postnatal blues, regaining one's waist, making up for lost sleep, learning to fit the housework into the baby's non-demanding spells, visiting the family planning clinic to plan the next baby, and generally settling down to a routine of family life' (Oakley 1981).

There is a growing body of evidence to support the notion that 'sadness' is indeed a normal part of women's postnatal experience as they grieve for their lost identity, lost control over their lives and unexpected changes in relationships (Nicolson 1990; McIntosh 1993; Barclay *et al* 1997; Podkolinski 1998). Oakley (1981) argues that this complex emotional reaction to motherhood is, rather than being a malfunction, a perfectly reasonable response that has two main origins: first, it is a response to the enormity of the change to women's social lives that motherhood brings in our culture, and second, it is a form of bereavement in which a woman mourns her former identity. Oakley suggests that the label 'depression' has been ascribed to the major legitimate strategy available to women for expressing the fact that the conditions of their lives are not congenial to them. The acknowledgement of 'sadness' as a normal part of women's feelings postnatally enables it to be perceived not as an individual's problem but as a public one for which society must take some responsibility.

This tension between the public expectations of women's experience of motherhood and their lived experience has been addressed by a number of writers. Rich (1978) makes the distinction between the public institution of motherhood and the private lived experience of mothering. According to her analysis, men have convinced women that unless a woman is a mother, she is not really a woman. In Oakley's analysis of women's experience of being a mother, good mothers are not supposed to have any personal friends, plans unrelated to those of their families, access to the public world, or their own wants and needs, are expected to be on the job 24 hours a day – yet they are supposed to be content (Oakley 1981). Rossiter, who undertook a phenomenological study of the transition into motherhood, observed: 'Women live a silent despair that comes from trying to respond to contradictory statements about mothering' (Rossiter 1988: 270).

■ Becoming a mother: childbirth as a rite of passage

The most fundamental change that occurs when a woman has a baby is that she becomes a mother. Contrary to the principles of the medical model, motherhood is not a temporary aberration that requires 'treatment' but a huge, profound and permanent transition in a woman's life. The intense significance of this, one of life's major transitions, must be set firmly at the centre of concern in maternity care by all who provide it:

> From onset to its destination, childbearing requires an exchange of a known self in a known world for an unknown self in an unknown world.
>
> (Rubin 1984)

Such a change in social role is characterised, in social terms, as a 'rite of passage'. Yearley (1997) explored birth as a rite of passage in a previous volume of this series. However, as childbirth is such an important transition in a woman's life, it is worth briefly revisiting this anthropological perspective of birth.

Davis-Floyd (1992) analyses birth as a rite of passage in American society. She uses van Gennep's (1966) definition of a rite of passage as:

> a series of rituals designed to conduct an individual (or group) from one social state or status to another, thereby effecting transformations both in society's perceptions of the individual and in the individual's perception of her- or himself.
>
> (Davis-Floyd 1992: 17)

There are three phases to a 'rite of passage':

- The 'rite of separation' from the old role;

- The 'liminal period' (a state of limbo between one social role and another);

- The 'rite of incorporation' as the individual adopts and is admitted into the new role.

Through interviews with women, midwives and obstetricians, Davis-Floyd explored the significance of the technocratic model of birth on American women's experience of birth. She concluded that the ritual use of high technology in pregnancy and birth denies the creative power of women. She offers many examples of how the rituals of technocratic birth deprive women of their 'cosmic significance as birth-givers, transformed in the transformation of giving birth into mere machines to be manipulated and repaired' (Davis-Floyd 1992: 286). Rituals are not required for 'transformations' to happen: the experience of labour and birth itself transfers the woman into the liminal situation. However, what the rituals do is to 'transmit' the core values of society to all participants in the birthing process. In British and American culture, these core values include the supremacy of technical and scientific knowledge and the subordinate status of women.

Women and midwives are perceived as being victims of this dominant belief system, which has eroded intuitive ways of knowing handed down from generation to generation and caused the loss of the women-centred rituals that in the past protected women from the exhaustion of childbirth. Contrast the following with the reality of many modern British women who go shopping in the supermarket only a few days after giving birth:

> The first week mother and child have to stay inside; a less restricted period of seclusion is supposed to last for 40 days from delivery. This is what happens in Africa, Asia and Latin America. The universal indigenous custom of keeping mother and child indoors is in accordance with the great vulnerability of both... as mother and child are believed to be

in a state of transition, they are considered to be very vulnerable to supernatural evil forces.

(Lefeber and Voorhoeve 1998: 51)

The postpartum period of childbirth is synonymous with the rite of incorporation, as the woman takes on her new role as mother. Seel (1986) and Yearley (1997) agree that the rite of incorporation is crucial to the rite of passage. If it is ignored, women are left 'high and dry' – the source of much unhappiness and distress. Some of the women's birth stories analysed in Davis-Floyd (1992) bear testimony to this, and the lack of supportive and protective postnatal 'rituals' for new mothers in the UK conveys the message that the culture in which we live does not value mothering. If postnatal care and thereby the experience of motherhood are to be improved for women, some fundamental beliefs and values about motherhood in our society and the role of the 'experts' need to be challenged. New 'rituals' need to be created that support and value new mothers.

Davis-Floyd demonstrates that when a woman's own experiences do not concur with the medical 'truth' about birth, she is left to feel a failure. Similarly, in Rossiter's study, women are shown to have only patriarchal discourses to draw on to explain their birth experiences: 'the only discourse available to Maria to explain why her birth preferences were ignored was "disappointment in her own body" – it must have been due to her own inadequacy' (Rossiter 1988: 275).

Rich's (1978) explanation for this phenomenon is that men fear women's mysterious powers and desire to control and contain the uncontrollable, thus maintaining their patriarchal authority. She argues that male doctors have devised rules for being pregnant and how to give birth – when and what to eat, how often to breastfeed and so on – but these rules frequently clash with women's lived experience. When this happens, a woman does not know whether to trust the authority of the doctors or the sensations and cues of her own body. This kind of experience transforms childbirth and motherhood into a profoundly alienating experience.

■ Authoritative knowledge

Another factor demonstrating the way in which women's lived experiences are discounted by the medical model is considered by Jordan (1993), who employs the concept of authoritative knowledge. She studied childbirth practices across a number of different cultures, observing how some types of knowledge hold more power than others 'regardless of "truth value"' (Jordan 1993: 149). For example, she analysed videotaped data of birth to demonstrate how technology and social interaction construct authoritative knowledge (Jordan 1997). She illustrates how women are not allowed to push spontaneously but only when an obstetrician has performed an examination and given his permission. She uses the dialogue between obstetric nurse, woman and obstetrician to illustrate clearly how there is a hierarchy of knowledge, priority being given to that of the obstetrician and the technology he employs. The woman's knowledge is dismissed (Jordan 1997).

In another study of village midwives and their medical trainers, Jordan observed that while in the training environment in hospital these midwives appeared to be 'stupid, illiterate, and inarticulate', in their home environment the knowledge and skills they had were respected (Jordan 1997: 60). She proposes that, in any social situation, some ways of knowing hold more legitimacy than others and devalue other knowledge. This Jordan terms 'authoritative knowledge'. Such knowledge may achieve authority because it is believed to be the 'truth', but it may also reflect the superior social power base of those who hold it. 'The devaluation of non-authoritative knowledge systems is one mechanism by which hierarchical social structures are generated, maintained, and displayed' (Jordan 1993: 152).

Bryar (1995), in her exploration of the models and theories that underpin midwifery practice, suggests that it is a practitioner's own beliefs and values that are fundamental to the model of care she adopts. 'Midwifery identifies clearly that the practice of midwifery is dependent on the use of *self* by the midwife' (Bryar 1995: 2). Thus midwives need to be able to develop and articulate their own beliefs and values about women and mothering in our society because these beliefs will be reflected in the care they give. If they give authority to a body of knowledge based on the medical model, they devalue the reality of the women for whom they care.

■ Women's reality

> It is the moment when she becomes a mother that a woman first confronts the full reality of what it means to be a woman in our society.
> (Oakley 1979: 1)

In a qualitative study following the experiences of 55 primigravid women, Barclay *et al* (1997) conveyed the enormity of the life changes experienced by women as they became mothers for the first time. As new mothers, they were forced to leave the adult, public, working world where their social life was theirs to control, where appointments could be made and kept, and in which day was day and night was night. The women described undergoing a profound change as they grappled with motherhood behind closed doors, feeling unprepared for the reality of life with a baby. Motherhood had not turned out to be what they had expected, and this perceived failure of realisation lowered their self-esteem and often led them to question their ability to be a good mother. This was followed by a readiness to 'have a go', but at the same time the women felt perpetually drained of both physical and emotional energy, alone and isolated, and held a sense of loss for their old way of life. However, by the end of this process, they reached a point where they had worked out a strategy for coping and felt more 'on top' of things, although the process of working it out involved huge compromise and often served only to emphasise their sense of loss and isolation from the world they once knew.

As practitioners, midwives are privy to an extraordinary amount of information about the reality of women's lives – we talk with and observe women on a daily basis – yet we have done little to incorporate this knowledge into our models of care. As Oakley (1981) writes, there remain considerable discrepancies between normal motherhood as typified by health professionals and normal motherhood as it is actually experienced by women. Knowledge about normal motherhood held by women themselves seems to be denied by professionals, even when directly confronted with it. The 'authoritative' body of knowledge about childbirth is the professional one, passed on to women by midwives – perhaps an expression of midwives' claim to status in the public, professional world (Kirkham 1996). The professionalisation of midwifery since the 1902 Midwives Act has been construed by several commentators to have created a barrier between the midwife and her clients (Kitzinger 1988; Kirkham 1996). Reid (1989: 223) observes that 'the cultural and epistemological gulf separating patients and biomedical professionals contrasts starkly with the shared values and understandings of traditional midwives and the women who seek their care'.

■ Listening to women

To understand the reality of women's feelings and experience of mother-hood, we need to ask, what is it like to become a mother in our society? What do women actually need to help them to adjust? Ball (1987) tried to rectify the persistence of the medical model in postnatal care when she explored women's reactions to motherhood and the role of postnatal care. She identified that lack of rest, sleep and social support were crucial to women's health, but her findings have made little impact on midwifery prac-tice (Marchant 1995).

However, in the 1990s, the work of systematically recording the experi-ence of childbearing women and using the findings to inform midwifery care is beginning. In Barclay's qualitative study, women identified three factors that appeared to mediate the process of becoming a mother: the baby's behaviour, social support and previous experience (Barclay *et al* 1997). Other studies have consistently demonstrated the desire of women for continuity and support, lots of support (Majewski 1987; Pridham & Zavoral 1988; Gjerdingen & Chaloner 1994). Stamp and Crowther (1994) found that the most helpful thing that women felt they were offered post-natally was emotional support, identified by over 50 per cent of women, *far* above any information or advice-giving, breastfeeding and babycare help, or physical care.

The value of social support during the postnatal period cannot be overestimated. Women derive enormous strength from knowing that other women share their doubts about their ability to be a good mother and feel similar feelings of loss and isolation (Podkolinski 1998). Women also learn skills and coping strategies from other experienced mothers and may gain comfort from knowing that they too felt completely at a loss in the early days. Sadly, the support that women receive from health professionals is not always viewed positively: many tales of conflicting advice persist, and too often a midwife's brisk competence in routine baby care tasks such as bathing and nappy-changing only serves to undermine even further a new mother's sense of her own inadequacy (Audit Commission 1997; Barclay *et al* 1997).

Prior to becoming mothers themselves, young women seldom have the opportunity to learn what to expect in the period of early motherhood in Western culture. One strategy suggested by the women in Barclay's study is for pregnant women to be given the opportunity to talk to experienced mothers, spend time with them and learn the coping strategies they have developed in order to prepare for their own impending motherhood. This is an approach that midwives might do well to explore. Certainly, women who have gained experience in handling small babies, either caring for their own siblings or working with children, seemed to be more prepared for the experience of becoming a mother (Barclay *et al* 1997).

The process of becoming a mother does not start in the postnatal period. Events during pregnancy and birth, most notably the presence or otherwise of support, have been shown to affect women's experience of motherhood. The provision of social support during pregnancy and one-to-one support during labour and birth has been shown to enhance a woman's positive feelings about being a mother and reduces her anxiety about the baby (Hodnett 1998).

Sadly, midwives are not trained to provide support. Their education, and the vast majority of their clinical experience, focuses even today on a medical approach to childbirth. Essential support skills such as facilitating groups, enabling discussion, listening and communicating, the use of touch, the use of the self as a therapeutic tool, and basic counselling techniques appear to be given a low priority in current midwifery education programmes. Given the importance that women ascribe to the provision of support throughout their childbearing experience, this imbalance should be addressed as a priority.

■ The importance of stories

Stories are a source of knowledge that has been displaced by the experts, who believe that they 'know better'. A consequence of the authority of scientific knowledge is that the value of women's own stories is diminished. However, one woman's personal story may have resonance for others, and sharing stories could be a vehicle for redefining motherhood as a public as well as a private matter. Midwives could help by facilitating this story-telling among women.

Kirkham (1997: 183) recognises the importance to women of their birth stories and the opportunity to tell them: 'A story tells more than its tale. It speaks of context and values.' Sharing stories helps women to give support to each other and aids understanding. The women in Podkolinski's (1998) study discovered this for themselves. Sharing their experience of early motherhood with other women facilitated a deeper understanding of the experience. It helped them not to feel alone, eased the guilt that they possessed about the baby, family and friends, and made them realise that it was not just their problem, to be sorted out alone.

The work of many female novelists, journalists and researchers testifies to the fact that women's experience of motherhood does not conform to their expectations, as well as documenting the extent to which society devalues the role of mothers (Rich 1978; Weldon 1981; Martin 1989; Karpf 1992; Walker 1992; Oakley 1993). Rossiter also used stories to explore women's experience of motherhood, following her own experience of becoming a mother. She wanted to understand 'how the way our society organises mothering helps to create the concept "Woman" as it exists in capitalist patriarchy' (Rossiter 1988: 11). Midwifery education programmes might like to explore the use of 'evidence' from the humanities about the realities of motherhood; women's writing could provide a rich resource for discussion and learning (Grant 1998).

■ The postnatal period

The imposition of an artificially defined postnatal period is another example of how the authoritative knowledge of the medical model bears little relationship to women's real lives. The postnatal period is currently defined as a period of not less than 10 and not more than 28 days after the end of labour, during which the continued attendance of a midwife is required (UKCC 1998). Yet problems clearly persist beyond 28 days, and input from health professionals after this time in the current system of care is minimal, health visitors focusing primarily on the growing baby. Equally, women take more than 28 days even to begin to articulate their own 'truth' about their experience of having a baby (Davis-Floyd 1992).

On the basis of their findings of extensive postnatal morbidity, Glazener *et al* (1993b) suggest redefining the length of the puerperium as 1 year. They suggest that attention be focused on devising measures to improve the help and advice that mothers receive during that time, such as strengthening the lay support organisations, extending maternity leave, introducing paternity leave, rescheduling the 6-week check to 3 or even 6 months, and enquiring at that time about common health problems. In truth, the length of time required to adapt to motherhood is likely to vary enormously between women. Bereavement workers know that the time to 'recover' from a significant loss is likely to be more than a year (Schuchter & Zisook 1993); if childbirth signifies the loss of one's known 'self', why should this be any less?

Yet asking a woman, however kindly, about tiredness, backache and depression is of little use unless there is help that can be offered, and current maternity care, with its emphasis on the medical model, may have little to offer. No 'cure' has yet been found for postnatal tiredness. Bowers (1985) found that 88 per cent of women dutifully attended their 6-week postnatal check-up, yet their health problems were seldom addressed to their satisfaction.

☐ What care do women want?

There are currently several studies researching new ways of providing post-natal care that might better address the needs of women as they have begun to be defined. These include a trial of a postnatal support pack and eight formal sessions of a postnatal support group (Reid 1997); up to 10 home visits from a postnatal support worker during the first 28 days (in addition to care from the community midwife) (Morrell *et al* 1997); and the use of a postnatal symptom checklist at 28 days, the current 6-week check being replaced by a midwifery consultation at 10–12 weeks after the birth (Bick *et al* 1997).

Yet it seems as though the first step is missing; we must first listen with our full attention to women's stories of how it is to be a new mother, and then let them tell us what care they would like from us. This is the only sure way to create a maternity service that is both needs led and woman centred.

☐ Two sides of postnatal care

Postnatal care cannot be considered in isolation. So much of what happens to women postnatally is related to events in pregnancy and during labour. Although women who have had normal deliveries experience long-term problems, morbidity is significantly increased with instrumental deliveries (Johanson *et al* 1993). The primary way by which a woman's postnatal experience will be improved is to ensure that all women receive a high standard of evidence-based care during pregnancy and birth. As part of effective postnatal care, health professionals need to work hard at reducing the 'cascade of intervention' (Inch 1982) that results in a high number of instrumental deliveries; suggestions for ways to do this have been well documented elsewhere (Rosser 1998).

■ Conclusion

Midwives need to clarify their aims and objectives for postnatal care. The sources of knowledge hitherto used to inform those aims and objectives have been drawn from medical literature and research. It has been recognised in the past 20 years that women have emotional and psychological needs in childbirth, but the service as it is currently organised is testimony to the fact that time and resources have not been allocated to meet those needs. We have seen how the medical model is not appropriate for supporting women through the transition into motherhood; yet most women give birth in a medical institution, and with a rising rate of instrumental and caesarean sections, an increasing number of women will need medical care to recover from the morbidity associated with their mode of birth. We cannot therefore abandon the medical model – this would be equally dishonest to women – but must combine it with an active social, cultural model that *does* contain the emotional supportive aspects that women have identified they need. Oakley (1993: 77) calls this provision of caring 'love'. She writes 'Love – caring – is as important as science – technical knowledge, monitoring and intervention – in the maternity services today'.

'Parenthood is a unique journey for each person who undertakes it' (Price 1988: 148). The postpartum period is often neglected, but midwives must recognise it as a crucial phase in the woman's journey through childbirth to motherhood and educate family and friends, indeed society generally, in how they can best support a woman and her partner at this time. Midwives can begin to record their extensive knowledge of women and the reality of mothering, and use their unique knowledge to help bring the social and cultural issues surrounding motherhood into the public domain to generate public and political debate.

Women need a new model of care that can accommodate the normal process of transition and change, which is not adequately addressed within the medical model. As discussed, the medical model becomes unstuck when it tries to medicalise normality. Midwives cannot cure a woman's backache postnatally or return her to the sexual being she was before she became a mother – the medical model has misled us here. What we need is a philosophy of caring that incorporates the medical model where appropriate and, for the rest and major part, embodies the 'being with' philosophy that is so much a part of midwifery. As midwives, it is both our task and our reward – to accompany women on their journey to motherhood. The first step is to listen to what they are telling us.

■ Recommendations for clinical practice in the light of currently available evidence

1. 'Becoming a mother' is one of the major rites of passage in a woman's life. An acknowledgement of the intense significance of this transition should be the focus of all midwifery care.

2. Becoming a mother is an irrevocable, profound and permanent change in a woman's life. Midwives should resist the temptation to fuel the myth that women will 'get back to normal' after giving birth.

3. Midwives should be aware of the limitations of the 'medical model' when dealing with normal childbirth, develop an understanding of other cultural, social and political factors that influence a women's well-being, and research ways of incorporating this understanding into their daily practice.

4. Midwives should be aware that their own personal beliefs, values and experiences of women, childbirth and motherhood influence the care that they give.

5. Midwives need to study and value sources of knowledge about childbirth other than just the authoritative knowledge of the 'medical model'. Studying women's experiences is a vital first step in this process.

6. Support consistently emerges from the literature as the component of postnatal care that women desire most. Midwives should actively help women to develop support networks to help them in their transition to motherhood, and should research the ways in which this support can best be provided.

7. If the maternity service is to respond to client need, the focus of midwifery education needs to shift towards educating student midwives to provide support to women throughout their childbearing careers.

■ Practice check

● Have you taken the time to listen to new mothers to find out what they are experiencing and what care they would like postnatally?

● List the good and bad things about being a mother in your culture. How might you respond to these factors in your own practice?

● Do you emphasise the importance of postnatal support with women and help them to devise strategies to organise the support they need? Are you aware of all the possible sources of postnatal support in your area?

● Do you offer a regular, ongoing postnatal support group to help women to talk to each other and share their experiences and skills? If not, could you set one up?

● What active steps do you take to help women to set up social support networks during pregnancy that will hopefully last into motherhood? Could you facilitate informal opportunities for primigravid women to talk to experienced mothers and possibly even to handle small babies?

● When you need to handle a baby, how might you do it in such a way as not to undermine a woman's confidence in and knowledge of her own baby?

- Does your midwifery team have a strategy in place to standardise information given to new mothers about common tasks such as infant feeding and sleeping, cord care and baby hygiene?

- How do you ensure that women make a genuine choice about whether they wish to receive a postnatal home visit on a certain day?

■ References

Audit Commission (1997) First Class Delivery: Improving Maternity Services in England and Wales. Audit Commission, London.

Ball JA (1987) Reactions to Motherhood: the Role of Postnatal Care. Books for Midwives Press, Hale.

Ball JA (1993) Physiology, psychology and management of the puerperium. In Bennett VR and Brown LK (eds) Myles' Textbook for Midwives, 12th edn. Churchill Livingstone, London, pp. 233–50.

Barclay L, Everitt L, Rogan F, Schmied V, Wyllie A (1997) Becoming a mother – an analysis of women's experience of early motherhood. Journal of Advanced Nursing, 25: 719–28.

Bick DE, MacArthur C (1995) The extent, severity and effect of health problems after childbirth. British Journal of Midwifery, 3(1): 27–31.

Bick D, MacArthur C, Winter H *et al* (1997) Redesigning postnatal care: physical and psychological needs. British Journal of Midwifery, 5(10): 621–2.

Bowers JP (1985) The six week postnatal examination. In Robinson S, Thomson AM (eds) Proceedings of the 1984 Research and the Midwife Conference. Nursing Research Unit, Kings College, University of London.

Bryar R (1995) Theories for Midwifery Practice. Macmillan, London.

Dalton K (1989) Depression after Childbirth, 2nd edn. Oxford University Press, Oxford.

Davis-Floyd RE (1992) Birth as an American Rite of Passage. University of California Press, Berkeley.

Dewan G, Glazener C, Tunstall M (1993) Postnatal pain: a neglected area. British Journal of Midwifery, 1(2): 63–6.

Garcia J, Marchant S (1996) The potential of postnatal care. In Kroll D (ed.) Midwifery Care for the Future. Baillière Tindall, London, pp. 58–74.

Gjerdingen DK, Chaloner K (1994) Mothers' experience with household roles and social support during the first postpartum year. Women and Health, 21(4): 57–74.

Glazener CMA (1997) Sexual function after childbirth: women's experiences, persistent morbidity and lack of professional recognition. British Journal of Obstetrics and Gynaecology, 104: 330–5.

Glazener C, Abdalla M, Russell I, Templeton A (1993a) Postnatal care: a survey of patients' experiences. British Journal of Midwifery, 1(2): 67–74.

Glazener CMA, MacArthur C, Garcia J (1993b) Postnatal care: time for a change. Contemporary Review of Obstetrics and Gynaecology, 5(3): 130–6.

Grant J (1998) Different ways of knowing. Practising Midwife, 1(11): 41.

Helman CG (1994) Culture, Health and Illness: An Introduction for Health Professionals, 3rd edn. Butterworth-Heinemann, Oxford.

Hodnett ED (1998) Support from caregivers during childbirth (Cochrane Review) In Cochrane Library, Issue 4, 1998, Update Software, Oxford.

Inch S (1982) Birthrights. Hutchinson, London.

Johanson R, Wilkinson P, Bastible A, Ryan S, Murphy H, O'Brien S (1993) Health after childbirth: a comparison of normal and assisted vaginal delivery. Midwifery, 9: 161–8.

Jordan B (1987) The hut and the hospital: information, power and symbolism in the artifacts of birth. Birth, 14(1): 36–40.

Jordan B (1993) Birth in Four Cultures. Waveland Press, Illinois.

Jordan B (1997) Authoritative knowledge and its construction. In Davis-Floyd RE, Sargent CF (eds) Childbirth and Authoritative Knowledge. University of California Press, Berkeley, pp. 55–99.

Karpf A (1992) Beyond belief. Guardian, 7 February, p. 29.

Kirkham M (1996) Professionalisation past and present: with woman or with the powers that be? In Kroll D (ed.) Midwifery Care for the Future. Baillière Tindall, London, pp. 164–201.

Kirkham M (1997) Stories and childbirth. In Kirkham MJ, Perkins ER (eds) Reflections on Midwifery. Baillière Tindall, London, pp. 183–204.

Kitzinger S (1988) Why women need midwives. In Kitzinger S (ed.) The Midwife Challenge. Pandora, London, pp. 1–20.

Lefeber Y, Voorhoeve H (1998) Indigenous Customs in Childbirth and Childcare. Van Gorcum, Assen, The Netherlands.

Limerick, Countess of (1939) Postnatal care. Journal of the Royal Institute of Public Health, 12: 358–67.

MacArthur C, Lewis M, Knox EG (1991) Health after Childbirth. HMSO, London.

McIntosh J (1993) Postpartum depression: women's help-seeking behaviour and perceptions of cause. Journal of Advanced Nursing, 18: 178–84.

Maclean G (1994) Safe motherhood: a basic right, or a privilege of a few? Modern Midwife, 6: 9.

Majewski J (1987) Social support and the transition to the maternal role. Health for Women International, 8: 397–407.

Marchant S (1995) What are we doing in the postnatal check? British Journal of Midwifery, 3(1): 34–8.

Martin E (1989) The Woman in the Body: A Cultural Analysis of Reproduction. Beacon Press, Boston.

Morrell CJ, Spiby H, Crowther S (1997) Postnatal social support: counting the cost. British Journal of Midwifery, 5(10): 613–15.

Nicolson P (1990) Understanding postnatal depression: a mother-centred approach. Journal of Advanced Nursing, 15: 689–95.

Oakley A (1979) From Here to Maternity: Becoming a Mother. Penguin, Harmondsworth.

Oakley A (1981) Normal motherhood: an exercise in self-control. In Hutter B, Williams G (eds) Controlling Women: The Normal and the Deviant. Croom Helm, London.

Oakley A (1993) Essays on Women, Medicine and Health. Basil Blackwell, Oxford.

Parr M, Whittaker V, Paden L (1997) Adaptation to parenthood and the new family. In Henderson C (ed.) Essential Midwifery. CV Mosby, London.

Podkolinski J (1998) Women's experiences of postnatal support. In Clement S (ed.) Psychological Perspectives on Pregnancy and Childbirth. Churchill Livingstone, Edinburgh, pp. 205–25.

Price J (1988) Motherhood – What it Does to Your Mind. Pandora, London.

Pridham KF, Zavoral JH (1988) Help for mother with infant care and household tasks: perceptions of support and stress. Public Health Nursing, 5(4): 201–8.

Reid M (1989) Sisterhood and professionalisation: A case study of the American lay midwife. In Shepherd McClain C (ed.) Women as Healers: Cross Cultural Perspectives. Rutgers University Press, London, pp. 219–38.

Reid M (1997) A randomised controlled trial of two interventions to provide social support. British Journal of Midwifery 5(10): 610–12.

Rich A (1978) Of Women Born. Virago Press, London.

Robinson J (1998) Dying for sex? Intercourse in the puerperium. British Journal of Midwifery, 6(11): 732–3.

Rosser J (1998) Caesarean sections: effective policies for risk management. Practising Midwife, 1(1): 9–10.

Rossiter A (1988) From Private to Public: A Feminist Exploration of Early Mothering. Women's Press, Toronto.

Rubin R (1984) Maternal Identity and the Maternal Experience. Springer, New York.

Schuchter SR, Zisook S (1993) The course of normal grief. In Stroebe MS, Stroebe W, Hansson RO (eds) Handbook of Bereavement: Theory, Research and Intervention. Cambridge University Press, Cambridge, pp. 23–43.

Seel R (1986) Birth rite. Health Visitor, 59(6): 182–4.

Silverton L (1993) The Art and Science of Midwifery. Prentice Hall International, Hemel Hempstead.

Stamp GE, Crowther CA (1994) Women's views of their postnatal care by midwives at an Adelaide Women's Hospital. Midwifery 10: 148–56.

Sweet BR (1997) Postnatal Care. In Sweet BR, Tiran D (eds) Mayes' Midwifery, 12th edn. Baillière Tindall, London, pp. 472–95.

Thomson AM (1996) Research into some aspects of postnatal care. In Robinson S, Thomson AM (eds) Midwives, Research and Childbirth, vol. 4. Chapman & Hall, London, pp. 208–37.

UKCC (1998) Midwives' Rules. UKCC, London.

Van Gennep A (1966) The Rites of Passage. University of Chicago Press, Chicago.

Walker A (1992) In Search of our Mothers' Gardens. Women's Press, London.

Weldon F (1981) Weekend. In Hill S (ed.) (1991) The Penguin Book of Modern Women's Short Stories. Penguin, Harmondsworth, pp. 352–71.

Woollett A, Dosanjh–Matwala N (1990) Postnatal care: the attitudes and experiences of Asian women in east London. Midwifery 6: 178–84.

Yearley C (1997) Motherhood as a rite of passage: an anthropological perspective. In Alexander J, Levy V, Roth C (eds) Midwifery Practice, Core Topics 2. Macmillan, London, pp. 23–37.

Chapter 2

The need to talk after birth: evaluating new services

Sally Marchant and Jo Garcia

■ Introduction

There has been a growing interest in providing women with the opportunity to discuss their birth experience, and many new initiatives have been set up to address this. In part, this is the result of an awareness that some women continue to have unresolved emotional distress linked to the birth. In addition, there is an increased appreciation that it is the woman's perception of the labour and birth, rather than how the birth is assessed by care-givers, that is of importance (Crompton 1996a, 1996b). In this chapter, we explore how these themes are related, considering the material under three headings:

- Women's varied needs for information and discussion about birth events;
- The current range of services being offered;
- The need for evaluation of what is being offered.

Figure 2.1 is intended to illustrate the linked topics that underpin this complex area.

■ It is assumed that you are already aware of the following:

- Current patterns of postnatal care;
- The range of psychological responses to major life events;
- The extent of postpartum psychological morbidity;
- The use of screening tools such as the Edinburgh Postnatal Depression Scale (Cox *et al* 1987);
- The debate about women's involvement in their care.

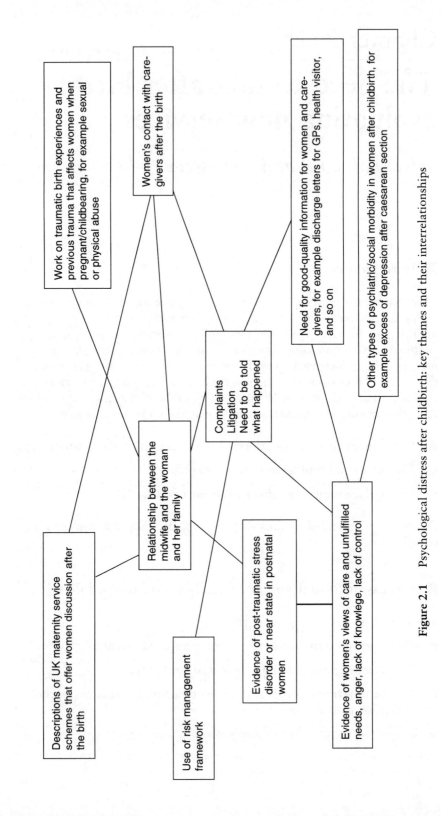

Figure 2.1 Psychological distress after childbirth: key themes and their interrelationships

■ Women's varied needs for information and discussion about the birth events

This is not an area that has been extensively researched, but there are some clues in studies of women's views of care and in anecdotal evidence about what women want. Women's needs vary widely. Many women have a general desire to talk about the birth to anyone who will listen. Others need quite specific information about birth events and implications for the future. Women may seek a respectful hearing or perhaps an apology when they feel that something has gone wrong. A few women may need counselling or psychiatric help because of continuing or unresolved distress.

There is a general awareness among maternity care-givers that, alongside the general desire to talk about the experience of the labour and birth (DiMatteo *et al* 1993), women may wish to clarify what happened or discuss the implications of pregnancy and birth events for future child-bearing. In a recent national postal survey of a representative sample of women who had given birth in June and July 1995 in England and Wales, one question asked whether they had been able to talk to a member of staff about their birth. Around one in five had wanted to do this but had not been able to (Garcia *et al* 1998). The questionnaire did not go into any detail about the topics that women would like to have discussed, but quite a number of women wrote comments in an open section at the end of the questionnaire, some of which are relevant to this issue. For example:

> In both my deliveries the reason for my having caesareans was explained to me by medical staff wearing masks and I was under the influence of epidurals. The information did not sink in. It would be nice to sit down with my GP who has my notes about four months later to talk about the delivery and future implications.

> I would have liked to discuss more why I was induced as was this the reason I had to have an emergency caesarean? I did ask the hospital doctor at my postnatal check but he was pretty non-committal. I also asked him if any future pregnancies would go the same way and he said I would probably need another caesarean, but didn't explain why.

We do not have evidence about what proportion of women have unmet needs for information after the birth, what type of information they need or when it is best for them to have it. Some may have been given the information, but at a time when they could not absorb it. On the other hand, women may find it hard to have their questions 'heard' by care-givers. There is evidence that encounters with care-givers often follow a pattern that is determined by the professional, with few opportunities for the woman to include the issues that are important to her. This is true of both doctors (see for example, Oakley 1979) and midwives (Kirkham 1989; Hunt & Symonds 1995; Lomax & Robinson 1996).

In practice, questions often arise when a couple are planning another pregnancy or when a woman is pregnant again. A study from over 20 years ago suggested that the need to make sense of the events of labour and birth can arise from gaps or 'missing pieces' in women's memories of events (Affonso 1977). Although a later study (Stolte 1986) could not replicate the findings of Affonso in full, it seems likely some women may be unable to remember certain aspects of their labour and the birth.

Where the woman or family feel that 'things went wrong', whether or not care would be objectively assessed as substandard, there is evidence to suggest that good communication and the opportunity to discuss events with relevant care-givers may make a difference, both to the feelings of the family and to the likelihood of formal complaints or litigation (Vincent *et al* 1994; Brown 1997; Symon 1997). However, listening to women when they have negative experiences of childbirth should not be based primarily on a desire to avoid litigation. We should be aware that good communication may lessen distress, especially where the woman may be blaming herself and where the events are associated with feelings of grievance. Women may have a need to have their experience acknowledged or to receive an apology. One woman in the Audit Commission (1997) survey wrote:

> I had to go back into hospital nine weeks after my baby was born to be re-cut and stitched... What annoyed me was the sister who stitched me... was there in the theatre when I was being re-stitched and I did not get an apology.

☐ More severe reactions

It is becoming clear, as a result of recent research, that there is only a scant understanding of the natural history and normal range of women's psychological health after childbirth. Women's own reports of their feelings after a difficult birth have been discussed by Sheila Kitzinger (1992), who drew attention to the similarity with feelings after a sexual assault. Recent studies have suggested that a small number of women may be suffering from full post-traumatic stress disorder (PTSD) or some post-traumatic stress reaction after gynaecological procedures (Menage 1993), miscarriage (Lee *et al* 1996) and caesarean section (Ryding 1997, 1998). PTSD is diagnosed using predetermined criteria (American Psychiatric Association 1994). Although it is now widely accepted that some women do suffer from PTSD after childbirth (Allen 1998; Lyons 1998), there is some debate in the literature about the criteria used to classify the condition (Crompton 1996a; Charles 1997; Hammett 1997). To date, studies in this area have been small. We need prospective studies of larger populations of women to look at the proportions with PTSD and related conditions, as well as at the main risk factors.

More information is also required about the links between depression following childbirth and severe states of anxiety or stress (Lyons 1998).

Although these are separate conditions, women with postnatal depression may also be suffering from emotional distress or PTSD (Lyons 1998). The treatment of postnatal depression with antidepressants, however, is unlikely to lead to a resolution of the emotional distress of PTSD.

Studies that have attempted to disentangle the symptoms displayed by women who have signs of psychological distress after childbirth are hampered by a lack of evidence to describe the range of normal feelings adequately. The emotional stages following bereavement have been described (see for example, Parkes & Weiss 1983), and it is possible that women who develop PTSD may have been left 'morbidly stuck' in a part of a process similar to grieving (H Allott, personal communication 1998). In one study of 20 women who had had traumatic childbirth experiences (Allen 1998), women who reported that they avoided thinking about the events and believed that they should not admit to difficulties in coping were more likely to continue to be distressed. In addition, it may be reasonable that women whose expectations have been shattered display anger and denial that they may be unable to resolve until they have information about the events.

In addition to women's reactions to the events of the birth itself, there is also the possibility that childbirth can act as a trigger to allow feelings related to pre-existing traumatic experiences to resurface (Rhodes & Hutchinson 1994; Lyons 1998). For example, women who have suffered sexual or other abuse may find that pregnancy or events around the birth bring back very painful feelings and memories (Rose 1992). Contact with care-givers may be difficult because physical examinations may be very frightening (J Kitzinger 1992). Care-givers have a difficult task in caring for women in this situation because the abuse may not be known either to the care-givers or, consciously, to the women themselves. On the other hand, sensitive care in the childbearing period may give abused women the opportunity to explore what has happened to them and find routes to recovery (Grant 1992).

In response to needs of the kind we have described, a wide variety of services are being set up, both within the NHS and by lay groups. It is these which we discuss next.

■ Current range of services being offered

It could be argued that routine midwifery practice already involves a discussion of the birth events, attempting to fill in any gaps in women's knowledge and to resolve queries and uncertainties. In some cases, the midwife who cared for the woman at the birth is the one to perform the function, while in other cases another midwife may ask about the birth during the course of postnatal care. This aspect of care is not normally made explicit, nor has it, as far as we know, been studied. For many midwives, however, making contact with the woman they have cared for, 1 or 2 days after the birth, is seen as common practice. Continuity of carer schemes should obviously make it much more likely that a woman will have the chance to talk about her birth with the midwife who cared for her at the time. This is borne out in the report of the evaluation of the One-to-One midwifery care scheme (McCourt & Page 1996), which showed that, in the main hospital covered by the study, 64 per cent of women cared for in the scheme had spoken to someone who had been present at the birth, compared with 19 per cent of women not in the scheme.

Explicit schemes have also been set up within the health service to offer women opportunities to talk about the birth. These schemes vary greatly. Some are offered to all women, while others are accessed by referral for women thought to have a problem that needs discussing. While some have been set up by midwives (Charles & Curtis 1994; Smith & Mitchell 1996), others are provided by obstetricians or mental health professionals.

In 1992, midwives in Winchester initiated a service that they called Birth Afterthoughts and invited women to contact them if they wished to talk about any of the events during the pregnancy, labour and childbirth (Charles & Curtis 1994). This arose largely as the result of an obstetric consultant receiving letters from women asking for details about their birth experiences. Women are invited to call an answerphone to leave their message. They are then contacted by a midwife, and an appointment is given. Women are seen on one occasion only for a maximum of 1.5 hours. During the meeting, the midwife has the mother's midwifery records available for discussion. The midwife completes a written summary of the visit, and the mother is invited to complete an anonymous questionnaire giving her views of the service. Other units have offered similar schemes.

In a similar way, arising from women's needs, a consultant obstetrician set up the Reading Post-delivery Stress Clinic, where women who have had distressing experiences can talk and be helped to plan for a future pregnancy or an impending delivery (Goldbeck-Wood 1996).

Outside the health service, lay groups in maternity care provide a range of places where women can discuss the birth. Postnatal groups may serve this function, among others. By having a telephone advice line, groups such as AIMS and the NCT often give women the chance to talk about their experiences and may refer women on to local contacts. Special services such as the Birth Crisis Network (Kitzinger 1998) allow women to discuss traumatic experiences with other women.

■ The need for an evaluation of what is being offered

There are recent articles recommending the routine offer of 'debriefing' without always being specific about what is meant (Crompton 1996b, Hammett 1997). In much of the literature, interventions are described as forms of debriefing without distinguishing between an agreed psychological treatment (Dyregrov 1989) and simply offering to listen to a woman's experiences and possibly explain any queries related to the birth. Concern has been expressed about this widespread use of the term 'debriefing' in the absence of any clear descriptions of what intervention is actually being used (Alexander 1998). The paper calls for greater clarity in the description, purpose and value of schemes associated with listening to women's experiences after childbirth. The author suggests that, while it might be difficult to imagine that the offer of an opportunity to talk through the birth could be harmful, there is as yet, without reliable evidence, no information about either the advantages or the disadvantages of such schemes. Similar points have been made by other writers (Raphael & Meldrum 1995; Waterson 1996).

Evaluation is needed because of the potential for interventions to do harm as well as good:

Good	Harm
● Less fear and anxiety	● Expectations that may not be met
● Greater confidence	● Opening painful issues
● A knowledge of events and implications	● Knowing when to refer
● Less anger and unhappiness	● Using resources that might be better used elsewhere
● Less litigation	

A recent review outside the maternity field of trials of debriefing (defined as a brief psychological intervention) for people who had suffered recent trauma suggested a harmful rather than a beneficial effect of the intervention (Wessely *et al* 1998). On the other hand, a small trial of a simple listening intervention for low-risk postnatal mothers carried out in Liverpool (Lavender & Walkinshaw 1998) appeared to show a beneficial effect on women's anxiety and depression at 3 weeks after delivery. In Australia, a trial that offers women a midwifery information and discussion session after caesarean section is nearing completion. Further evaluation of the wide range of interventions that are intended to prevent distress is clearly needed. Studies should explore:

● The types of intervention for postnatal women;

● The person who offers such interventions;

● Whether training is necessary, and if so, of what type;

● The time, place and setting for any intervention.

Two other areas could also be explored. The first is whether attempting to give women information antenatally that might make their expectations more 'realistic' could improve their psychological outcome. This is based on the finding that some women suffered distress if their labour was very different from what they had expected (Allen 1998; Lyons 1998). Second, it might be useful to look at information-giving after the birth in relation to specific issues such as the need for subsequent caesarean section, or the likelihood that a particular problem will recur. This information could be provided to women and also to the primary care-givers, who are likely to see them after the birth and advise them if they consider another pregnancy. In addition, we need to collaborate with psychologists and psychiatrists to evaluate different treatments for PTSD and other forms of distress.

■ Conclusion

This is just one example of an area where care-givers and lay groups create innovative services in response to women's needs. This desire to respond to perceived shortcomings in the care they are providing is at the core of the caring professions. At the same time, there is a risk that care can be ineffective or even harmful. Maternity services are increasingly willing to adapt what they do while evaluating the changes. This shows a confidence in the power of research to support and develop practice.

■ Recommendations for clinical practice in the light of currently available evidence

1. It is important that the organisation of midwifery care allows midwives to have time to listen actively to what women have to say.

2. The profession needs to consider how to 'raise the status' of what women have to say about their birth experience; women could be invited to write or dictate an account to be kept with their notes.

■ Practice check

● How do you make time to listen to what women in your care have to say about their experiences of motherhood?

● If you have been involved with a birth, do you try to see the woman again postnatally?

● Have you had any training in counselling?

● What are the referral mechanisms for women who are psychologically distressed?

● Do you have the telephone numbers for the relevant support groups?

■ References

Affonso DD (1977) Missing pieces – a study of postpartum feelings. Birth, 4(4): 159–64.

Alexander J (1998) Confusing debriefing and defusing postnatally: the need for clarity of terms, purpose and value. Midwifery, 14(2): 122–4.

Allen SA (1998) A qualitative analysis of the process, mediating variables and impact of traumatic childbirth. Journal of Reproductive and Infant Psychology, 16(2/3): 107–31.

American Psychiatric Association (1994) Anxiety disorders: post traumatic stress disorder. In Diagnostic and Statistical Manual of Mental Disorders, 4th edn. American Psychiatric Association, Washington, pp. 424–9.

Audit Commission (1997) First Class Delivery: Improving Maternity Services in England and Wales. Audit Commission, London.

Brown C (1997) Someone to blame. New Generation (Jun): 7.

Charles C (1997) When the dream goes wrong... post-traumatic stress disorder. Midwives, 110(1317): 250–2.

Charles J, Curtis L (1994) Birth afterthoughts – setting up a listening service. Midwives Chronicle, 107(1278): 266–8.

Cox JL, Holden JM, Sagovsky R (1987) Detection of postnatal depression. Development of the 10-item Edinburgh Postnatal Depression Scale. British Journal of Psychiatry, 150: 782–6.

Crompton J (1996a) Post-traumatic stress disorder and childbirth. British Journal of Midwifery, 4(6): 290–3.

Crompton J (1996b) Post-traumatic stress disorder and childbirth: 2. British Journal of Midwifery, 4(7): 354–5, 373.

DiMatteo MR, Kahn KL, Berry SH (1993) Narratives of birth and the postpartum: analysis of the focus group responses of new mothers. Birth, 20(4): 204–11.

Dyregrov A (1989) Caring for helpers in disaster situations: psychological debriefing. Disaster Management, 2(1): 25–30.

Garcia J, Redshaw M, Fitzsimons B, Keene J (1998) First Class Delivery: A National Survey of Women's Views of Maternity Care. Audit Commission, London.

Goldbeck-Wood S (1996) Post–traumatic stress disorder may follow childbirth. British Medical Journal, 313: 774.

Grant E (1992) Effects of childhood sexual abuse: issues for obstetric caregivers. Birth, 19(4): 220–1.

Hammett PL (1997) Midwives and debriefing. In Kirkham MJ, Perkins ER (eds) Reflections on Midwifery. Baillière Tindall, London, pp. 135–59.

Hunt S, Symonds A (1995) The Social Meaning of Midwifery. Macmillan, Basingstoke.

Kirkham M (1989) Midwives and information-giving during labour. In Robinson S, Thomson A (eds) Midwives, Research and Childbirth, vol. 1. Chapman & Hall, London, pp. 117–38.

Kitzinger J (1992) Counteracting, not re-enacting, the violation of women's bodies: the challenge for perinatal caregivers. Birth, 19(4): 219–20 .

Kitzinger S (1992) Birth and violence against women: generating hypotheses from women's accounts of unhappiness after childbirth. In Roberts H (ed.) Women's Health Matters. Routledge, London, pp. 63–80.

Kitzinger S (1998) Just when you thought it was all over... New Generation (Sep): 16–17.

Lavender T, Walkinshaw SA (1998) Can midwives reduce postpartum psychological morbidity: a randomized trial. Birth, 25(4): 215–19.

Lee C, Slade P, Lygo V (1996) The influence of psychological debriefing on emotional adaptation in women following early miscarriage: a preliminary study. British Journal of Medical Psychology, 69(1): 47–58.

Lomax H, Robinson K (1996) Asymmetries in interaction: an analysis of midwife–client talk during the postnatal period. In International Confederation of Midwives, 24th Triennial Conference, Oslo May 1996. International Confederation of Midwives, London, pp. 252–5.

Lyons SA (1998) Prospective study of post traumatic stress symptoms 1 month following childbirth in a group of 42 first-time mothers. Journal of Reproductive and Infant Psychology, 16(2/3): 91–105.

McCourt C, Page L (1996) Report on the Evaluation of One–to–One Practice. Hammersmith Hospitals NHS Trust and Thames Valley University, London.

Menage J (1993) Post-traumatic stress disorder in women who have undergone obstetric and/or gynaecological procedures. A consecutive series of 30 cases of PTSD. Journal of Reproductive and Infant Psychology, 11: 221–8.

Oakley A (1979) Becoming a Mother. Martin Robertson, Oxford.

Parkes CM, Weiss RS (eds) 1983 Recovery from Bereavement. Basic Books, New York.

Raphael B, Meldrum L (1995) Does debriefing after psychological trauma work? British Medical Journal, 310(6993): 1479–80 (editorial).

Rhodes N, Hutchinson S (1994) Labor experiences of childhood sexual abuse survivors. Birth, 21(4): 213–20.

Rose A (1992) Effects of childhood sexual abuse on childbirth: one woman's story. Birth, 19(4): 214–8.

Ryding EL, Wijma B, Wijma K (1997) Post-traumatic stress reactions after emergency caesarean section. Acta Obstetrica et Gynecologica Scandinavica, 76(9): 856–61.

Ryding EL, Wijma K, Wijma B (1998) Predisposing psychological factors for post-traumatic stress reactions after emergency cesarean section. Acta Obstetrica et Gynecologica Scandinavica, 77(3): 351–2.

Smith JA, Mitchell S (1996) Debriefing after childbirth: a tool for effective risk management. British Journal of Midwifery, 4(11): 581–6.

Stolte K (1986) Postpartum 'missing pieces': sequela of a passing obstetrical era? Birth, 13(2): 100–3.

Symon A (1997) Midwives and litigation. Improving communication: apologies and explanations. British Journal of Midwifery, 5(10): 594–6.

Vincent C, Young M, Phillips A (1994) Why do people sue doctors? A study of patients and relatives taking legal action. Lancet, 343(8913): 1609–13.

Waterson P (1996) Debriefing following childbirth: is it effective? MA News, 15: 5–6.

Wessely S, Rose S, Bisson J (1998) A systematic review of brief psychological interventions ('debriefing') for the treatment of immediate trauma related stress symptoms and the prevention of post traumatic stress disorder (Cochrane Review). In Cochrane Library, Issue 3. Update Software, Oxford.

Chapter 3

Perinatal grief: understanding the bereaved and their carers

Rosemary Mander

■ Introduction

Our understanding of the carer's painful grief associated with the loss of a baby has markedly increased since Bourne's research drew attention to our medical colleagues' difficulties when facing such a death (1968). Those midwives with long memories remember that medical personnel were not alone in encountering such difficulty. Midwives found themselves resorting to the 'rugger pass' approach to cope with caring for the bereaved mother (Mander 1994).

In this chapter, research is used to examine the personal implications of childbearing loss, including staff reactions, as illustrated by a case study. The focus is first on the parents bereaved through stillbirth or miscarriage. Next, the research that has provided this information and thus increased our understanding of childbearing loss will be discussed. In the third section, we will return to the research into the personal implications of emotionally traumatic experiences by considering studies of the effects on those who process the research data; this involves mainly the costs to the researcher and/or data collector. Then the strategies that have been used by researchers to assist their coping with emotionally challenging situations will be scrutinised. An attempt is made to relate the coping strategies that help the researcher to the midwife's role when providing care in situations of loss. Finally, we will contemplate the extent to which these researchers' coping strategies are relevant to the midwife caring for the grieving mother or parents.

■ It is assumed that you are already aware of the following:

● The ways in which a mother during her pregnancy comes to know and love her baby (the term 'baby' rather than 'fetus' will be used because this is how the mother regards her pregnancy from early on (Lumley 1980);

- The links between human attachment, or love, and the grief that is experienced if a valued and/or loving relationship ends;

- The processes and activities that a person utilises when she grieves the loss of someone who is loved or something on which she has depended (Robinson & McKenna 1998);

- The care that is ordinarily provided for a mother grieving a baby who has died or been miscarried (Mander 1994);

- The extent to which emotional support has been shown to facilitate healthy grieving (Kalish 1985).

■ Grief

Grief has historically been regarded as a less than positive phenomenon (Pine & Brauer 1986), but this view appears to be changing. The result is that grief, although it may occasionally develop into a pathological state (Rynearson 1987), now tends to be perceived as a healthy and necessary reaction. Grief has been defined as 'a normal, dynamic individualised process which pervades every aspect (physical, emotional, social, spiritual) of persons experiencing the loss' (Jacob 1993: 1789). Grief helps a person to cope with or adjust to the loss of a loving relationship or one that she has valued in another way.

□ Grief reactions and perinatal grief

Assumptions are often made about the process of grieving and may originate in any of a number of sources, sometimes being research based. Reactions following a night club fire (Lindemann 1944), the grief that follows a husband's death (Parkes 1972; Stroebe & Stroebe 1987) and that of the person approaching death (Kübler-Ross 1970) are examples of grief research. These studies have facilitated our understanding of the processes by which people work through the trauma of an event that might have been unthinkable, even unbearable. The extent to which they have informed our understanding of the loss of a baby is, however, less certain.

We have long known that grieving is not straightforward (Stroebe & Stroebe 1987) and that it varies between individuals. The tortuous journey through grief manifests itself in oscillation, hesitation and, hopefully, progress. Additionally, although supposedly normal grieving involves many challenges, grieving also carries the risk of becoming pathological. This has been attributed either to something preventing its onset or causing delay, or to difficulty completing the 'grief work', which results in the grieving becoming prolonged.

Recent research into perinatal grief reactions has suggested that the picture is even less clear than was previously assumed. An authoritative study by Lin and Lasker (1996) suggests that the onset and progress of perinatal grief is affected by a range of personal factors. The sample included 163 women, and 56 of their partners, who were bereaved through miscarriage, stillbirth or neonatal death. As with most grief research, the attrition rate was high: only 122 parents (55.7 per cent) completed all three interviews. The analysis of these parents' grief scores over the 2 years following their loss showed four patterns of grieving:

- In 41.0 per cent of parents, there was a steady decline in the grief score. This was described as a 'normal' pattern and was associated with being the mother and with a subsequent successful pregnancy.

- In 13.1 per cent of parents, the grief scores increased; these parents were referred to as the 'reversed' grief group. In this group, there was a low proportion of previous pregnancy loss and a high proportion of subsequent pregnancy loss.

- The 'delayed' resolution group comprised 17.2 per cent of parents. At the first interview, they had relatively low scores, but by the second interview the grief score was highest. This group had the highest proportion of late pregnancy loss and previous loss.

- The fourth group, the 'low' unchanged group, which showed grief scores that remained steady and low throughout the study, consisted of 28.7 per cent of the parents. This group comprised a larger proportion of fathers and had a larger number of children when the loss happened.

This study reminds us of the long-term nature of grief and the many factors that affect it, one of which is the gender of the parent. The manifestation of grief or mourning behaviour has been shown to differ between mothers and fathers (Dyregrov 1991; Cordell & Thomas 1997), but the association between gender and the grief underpinning that mourning is unclear.

Lin and Lasker's work suggests that the father's grief was not as intense as the mother's and that the men's feelings did not change over the 2-year period. These findings are supported by a large study of men whose partners experienced a miscarriage (Beutel *et al* 1996). It found that the father's grief is both less intense and less enduring than the mother's. In contrast, a Dutch study found that, among couples grieving the loss of a baby with a major congenital abnormality, the parents grieved in ways that were not significantly different (Hunfeld *et al* 1996). This finding of similarity between the grieving of the parents also emerged in a UK study of the grief reactions of the partners of women who miscarried (Johnson & Puddifoot 1996). The men's grief was influenced by the stage of the pregnancy at which the miscarriage occurred and also by whether the father had been with the mother when she had an ultrasound scan, both 'seeing' the baby then. This complex picture of male grief is further informed by Worth's qualitative study of men grieving a stillborn child (1997). Worth suggested that the demands on men are aggravated, and their grieving made more difficult, by their expectation that they assume a fathering role; this role includes activities such as 'acknowledging the child's reality', 'incorporating the child into the family' and 'maintaining memories' (1997: 78). Thus, conflicting personal and societal expectations impede not only men's mourning behaviour, but also their grieving.

So, although research exists in these areas, it is still not clear how the degree of attachment with the baby influences grief and whether it affects parents differently. I consider below whether and how the 'voluntariness' of the loss and the gestation of the fetal demise may affect the parental reaction.

Just as mothers' and fathers' grieving patterns and mourning behaviours vary, so different ethnic groups' mourning rituals also differ (Bartos & Mander 1995). The extent to which mourning reflects different grieving patterns among various cultures was researched by Cowles (1996). This study comprised several focus groups involving people from specific cultural backgrounds. Cowles showed that mourning behaviour did vary but that the personal experience of grief did not differ in any way that could be attributed to cultural heritage or ethnicity alone.

It has been assumed that because a relationship ends after a shorter period, there is less emotional investment and grief (Iles 1989); this may explain the limited significance traditionally attached to miscarriage by health care providers. This assumption has been questioned by recent research such as a prospective study involving 459 women, half of whom had recently experienced a miscarriage and the remainder of whom had not been pregnant within the preceding year (Neugebauer *et al* 1997). The risk of a serious emotional disorder, such as depression, was 2.5 times more likely to affect the women who had miscarried compared with the control group. A review of the psychological literature showed that, following miscarriage, a woman is likely to present with symptoms of a grief reaction (Frost & Condon 1996). These authors identify unique characteristics of grief following miscarriage, including guilt, feelings of a lost body part and a changed personal identity. This picture of postmiscarriage grief is endorsed by Lee and Slade (1996), who compare miscarriage with other forms of trauma and suggest that similar therapeutic interventions should be available.

The couple whose baby dies neonatally have been said to experience a healthier grief reaction as a result of the care and time that are invested by neonatal staff in the care of both them and their baby (Farnsworth 1996). This anecdotal observation was tested retrospectively through semi-structured interviews with 19 couples who had lost a baby through either intrauterine death (IUD) or through neonatal death (NND) (Schaap *et al* 1997). The grieving of the IUD parents had not progressed as well as those in the NND group. This was apparent in the IUD parents' difficulty in sharing or discussing their loss, more likely to be grieving 'discongruently' and more likely to be experiencing emotional and/or psychosocial problems.

Because it is a form of care that is becoming increasingly familiar, carers in general may make assumptions about the intensity of grief following the termination of a pregnancy. The effect of intentionality was studied using five well-validated instruments to measure, on four occasions over 1 year, the psychological state of two groups of women who had lost a pregnancy (Salvesen *et al* 1997). One group comprised women whose pregnancy had been terminated following the identification of congenital abnormalities by ultrasound scan (TOPFA group). The other group had lost a baby through late miscarriage, stillbirth or early NND. The researchers found that, in terms of their grief reactions, the only difference was that the TOPFA group reported significantly milder symptoms in the early days. This group was also found by 12 months to be significantly more likely to have been trying to start another pregnancy. Unable to attach any meaning to these differences, Salvesen *et al* conclude that intentionality does not affect perinatal grieving.

☐ Researching perinatal grief

If the midwife or other carer is to provide an environment in which grief may proceed healthily, she needs to utilise research findings such as those discussed above. Should she omit to use the research evidence, her care may have an effect other than that which she seeks. As Chalmers (1993) reminds us, a crucial prerequisite to using research is a critical reading of research literature to ensure that the evidence is strong enough to support our practice. We will now examine the methods that have been employed to study care following childbearing loss. This examination not only demonstrates the relevance of research to midwifery practice and the strength of that research, but also leads us to consider the more personal costs associated with researching perinatal loss and, eventually, to the vulnerability of the midwife who provides care. Following Chalmers' recommendation, we will begin this review with those methods which are more objective and scientific, and are sometimes assumed to provide stronger evidence (Gribben 1998).

The postal questionnaire was the data collection instrument for a nationwide epidemiological survey in Sweden (Rådestad *et al* 1996). As research texts remind us, postal questionnaires are suitable for collecting data from a large number of respondents over a wide geographical area at minimal cost (Rees 1997: 81). Unfortunately, convenience may be counter-balanced by low response rates and the superficial nature of the data. Rådestad *et al* sent the questionnaire to all Swedish women who had given birth to a stillborn baby in 1991 and to an equivalent control group with a live child: the response rate for study and control groups was high, being 83 per cent and 85 per cent respectively and producing 636 responses. Like many written questionnaires, these researchers' instrument included a large proportion of closed items; however, the data do illuminate or 'inform' the experience of the bereaved mother. The questionnaire probed topics such as 'meeting' the baby, creating memories and emotional support. A Likert-type scale was used to probe aspects such as ascertaining whether 'staff showed respect/tenderness to my child' and 'the delivery is a pleasant memory'.

Following their survey, these researchers identified a difficult issue relating to how much the midwife should encourage the mother to 'meet' or make contact with her baby. This problem was raised by 'Bessie', a midwife whom I interviewed during my study of the midwife's care of the woman who does not have her baby with her. She talked to me about this difficult decision:

> I'd never force anyone, though. I certainly would not want to cuddle anything that was dead myself.
>
> (Mander 1994: 62)

Rådestad *et al* also found that the mothers regarded properly taken photographs as essential to healthy grieving. This is a finding that carries serious organisational implications, especially for the purchase of equipment and the education of midwives, but that may also cause some clinical difficulty as shown in the case study below.

Another example of a postal questionnaire shows that their disadvantages may be greater than those found in the Swedish study. In the study by Prendiville *et al* (1997), a single-shot questionnaire was posted to 500 GPs to examine early miscarriage care in Ireland. Despite a response rate of 39 per cent, these researchers recommended that the GP is the ideal person to initiate care and that access to ultrasound would further improve management. We have to question, as there is no way of knowing, whether the 61 per cent of the sample who did not respond would endorse or even agree with this recommendation.

The randomised controlled trial (RCT) has become the 'gold standard' by which the effectiveness of care is assessed (Cochrane 1972). While a gut reaction may be that such a 'hard-edged' approach could not appropriately study an area as sensitive as bereavement care, Forrest *et al* (1982) showed that this is not so. These researchers' RCT lasted 18 months and recruited 50 women who had lost babies at 28 weeks' gestation or later. Of these women, equal numbers had given birth to stillborn babies and to liveborn babies who died neonatally. The women were randomly allocated to either 'routine care' or 'planned support'; the latter (experimental) group experienced 'ideal' care, which comprised being offered bereavement counselling and other interventions to facilitate healthy grieving. Whereas the minimum standard of care for the routine care group applied in only a 'few' cases, the researchers omit to mention how many of the 'ideal care' group actually accepted the interventions under scrutiny.

Data collection at 6 and 14 months was through semi-structured interviews with an interviewer 'blind' to the women's care group, together with self-completion of two well-validated instruments to identify mental health problems. Difficulty with follow-up resulted from some women refusing further participation and some GPs wishing to avoid 'upsetting' parents; thus, the response rate had fallen to 60 per cent by 14 months. Despite this, social isolation and a lack of intimate supportive relationships were found to be associated with a higher prevalence of mental health problems. In terms of resolving their grief, the supported mothers recovered more quickly than their counterparts who had routine care. The researchers assume that shorter grief is healthier, but the basis of this assumption is uncertain. This RCT indicated the value of midwifery support for a bereaved woman. Although this study encountered the problems often associated with grief research, such as high attrition rates (Leon 1990), the findings are endorsed by a Dutch study on a sample who had experienced one type of loss (Hunfeld *et al* 1997).

Another RCT focused on routine psychotherapeutic counselling following perinatal loss and also demonstrates sampling problems (Lilford *et al* 1994). Of 127 eligible couples, only 72 (57 per cent) agreed to participate, of whom 15 were referred directly for counselling and 57 were randomised. Additionally, unbalanced randomisation resulted in the study group comprising 35 couples (plus 15 direct referrals) compared with only 22 control couples. The outcome in terms of recovery from grief showed no difference between the treated and the untreated group. The first author criticises the intervention, concluding that the mothers who attended for counselling would probably have resolved their grief more satisfactorily anyway.

Lilford's criticism of counselling is endorsed by the findings of a North American study (Thomas & Striegel 1995) that moves our examination of the methods used to research grief away from the objective towards more qualitative approaches. These researchers assessed parents' coping abilities by interviewing 26 couples who had, within the previous 2 weeks, lost a baby through miscarriage or stillbirth. They used methodological triangulation to integrate qualitative and quantitative approaches and found that there were immense coping resources within the relationship on which the couple could draw. Data on the interaction within each relationship were collected by questionnaire, the completion of which was followed by a 3-hour semi-structured interview. The analysis of the ethnographic interview data demonstrated that the couple's emotional resources were more than adequate and that they shared understanding and common coping strategies. Additionally, the quantitative data showed their plentiful coping skills.

The pioneering work of Gohlish (1985) moves our scrutiny of research methods towards qualitative approaches, although her data collection comprised interview and 'Q sort', a numerical ranking technique. This exploratory study illuminated the previously underresearched area of women's perceptions of midwifery care and was undertaken by a midwife at a time when childbearing loss was still widely ignored. Gohlish contacted 15 out of 21 eligible women who had given birth to a stillborn baby in one maternity unit during a given year, and interviewed them at 10–42 days postnatally. Although this sample seems small, the response rate (71 per cent) compares well with that of other studies. The 'Q sort' technique involved signifying agreement or otherwise by weighting 30 specially prepared statements. The areas that were covered in Gohlish's statements related to emotional support, facilitating grieving and promoting physical comfort postnatally. This research demonstrated the importance that grieving women attach to assuming control over a seemingly uncontrollable situation.

A scrutiny of research methods in the area of childbearing loss suggests that qualitative approaches (Moulder 1998) may be appropriate. Moulder's Department of Health-funded study sought a systematic account of women's experiences and staff's subjective experience of providing care. The data were collected first by interviewing 20 women who had recently given birth to a stillborn baby or had experienced a miscarriage or termination of pregnancy. Second, these women were asked to keep a diary. Interviews were held with 70 staff from a range of grades and occupations. The interviews' semi-structured format 'allowed free interaction between the researcher and the interviewee and the opportunity to uncover areas previously not considered' (1998: 236). It is unfortunate that details of the methods and data analysis are scanty, and the use of 'predetermined headings' to collate the interview data (1998: 240) casts doubt on the study's qualitative credentials. The reluctance of qualitative researchers to detail their data analysis is a not uncommon problem (Nolan & Hicks, 1997: 182); this may aggravate the widespread misconception that qualitative research is more simplistic, and the data less authoritative, than research involving numerical analyses.

Rajan (1994) reports an intervention study that constituted the qualitative component of a large RCT. The intervention comprised midwifery support to women with a 'high-risk' pregnancy. Data were collected by interview between the research midwives and 84 previously bereaved mothers. This study suggests that bereaved women may be unable to find the emotional support that might be expected from their family and friends. Unlike Thomas and Striegel (1995), the male partner was found to experience loss in his own way and was unlikely to share the mother's need to articulate her loss or express it in other ways. Rajan identified how the need for the grieving mother to support her partner and significant others resulted in her delaying her own grieving, observing: 'the woman put everyone's needs before her own' (1994: 98). In this way, Rajan showed that the mother, whose need is greatest, lacks support while she is supporting others. Additionally, people whom the mother had previously regarded as friends were unable to cope with social contact with her after her bereavement, so erstwhile friends avoided contact to the extent of literally crossing the road to avoid speaking to her. Thus, Rajan's work highlights the grieving mother's need for an everyday sort of social contact with the usual range of people.

The research that I undertook into the midwife's care of a particularly vulnerable group of grieving mothers illuminates the midwife's decision-making in this situation (Mander 1991). A phenomenological design was adopted, this choice being based on the need to understand the experience of both being cared for and providing care. Additionally, previous researchers in this area – relinquishment for adoption – had encountered considerable difficulty in using a survey (Burnell & Norfleet 1979). Despite generous funding from the Iolanthe Trust, I decided that, by being the sole researcher/interviewer, I would gain deeper and more meaningful insights into the experiences of the women and the midwives who were interviewed. The fieldwork with the mothers comprised mainly retrospective accounts of their care and of relinquishment for adoption from women who had previously relinquished. The research design, however, incorporated an attempt to follow a woman prospectively through her experience of relinquishment. This prospective account, comprising both interviews and observation, formed the basis of a case study that provided the opportunity to check on the extent to which the previously relinquishing mothers' retrospective accounts still pertained. Each midwife gave me her impressions of the similarities between the care that she provides for the relinquishing mother and for the bereaved mother (Mander 1995).

This examination of the research methods used to investigate loss in childbearing has been moving in the direction of the researcher being increasingly involved with the research and the informants. The ultimate example of involvement is found in Farnsworth's study (1996), which shows the strengths of the researcher's deep personal and emotional input. Farnsworth used her personal experience, of being the mother of a small baby who died, to facilitate her research interaction with grieving mothers. Using family stress theory and feminist theory as her theoretical framework, Farnsworth used a reflexive format to interview all of the 10 mothers in depth for about 5 hours each. Her own experience of grieving her child's death 'guided' her research planning and data collection. In her interviews with grieving mothers, Farnsworth illustrates her intimate involvement by reporting how she was listening to herself as well as to the mother-informant. An important finding that emerged from this study, and supports that of Rajan (1994), is the caution that the bereaved mother learns regarding her ability to 'share her feelings' (1996: 401). Each mother in Farnsworth's study reported how friends and family had 'marginalised' her experience of loss. This caution resulted in each mother being relieved to learn that the researcher had been through a similar experience and was more likely to understand her perspective. That the mother is generally regarded as passive rather than a 'creative actor' following her loss also emerges from Farnsworth's work (1996: 409), which resonates with Gohlish's findings (1985). According to Farnsworth, none of the women regarded herself as passive, each having redefined herself to become more assertive in her work, family and social contexts.

☐ The personal costs

My own experience of interviewing mothers who had relinquished a baby and midwives who cared for grieving mothers persuaded me that the personal costs to the researcher may be great (Mander 1995). Clinical experience, as detailed in the case study below, convinces me that this may also be true for the midwife who provides care for a bereaved mother. However, the personal implications for the researcher are largely unmentioned and may be unmentionable (Brannen 1988), which may also apply to the midwife. While certain that I am not unique in finding such intimate contact with sorrow challenging to my coping skills, I have been able to locate little mention of such difficulties in the literature relating to either researchers or practitioners.

The existence of, and reason for, this longstanding neglect of the researcher in the literature has been observed and explained by Freilich (1979) in relation to anthropologists working in isolated settings. Freilich admits that research projects encounter difficulties but maintains that such an admission is unusual because 'the anthropological community... has provided only minimal encouragement to publish on methods and field experiences' (1979: 26–7). He explains that writing up 'these painful experiences' is not a priority, and the material becomes irrelevant through age.

This reluctance to admit to experiencing difficulty is fostered by the 'anthropological community', which discusses only positive aspects of fieldwork. Freilich observes that 'it is rare indeed to hear a speaker describe the emotional pains of field work' (1979: 27). He suggests that the memories of pain, anxiety and sorrow become subsumed beneath the other research demands. This process, which eventually anaesthetises the researcher to the pain, is assisted by ascribing any difficulties to 'personal incompetence' (1979: 27). Whether this anaesthesia is deliberate, Freilich is uncertain, but he recognises 'self-deception' as a coping strategy.

Unlike Freilich, Gans (1982) discusses the researcher's difficulty, but it is in the context of maintaining the participant observer's role and the necessary deception. Gans emphasises the tensions arising out of retaining a suitable emotional distance from informants, associated with ensuring the researcher's academic objectivity, and ensuring a consistently neutral stance.

These researchers' observations are sadly familiar. Freilich's account reinforces the 'myth of the perfect project', which engenders profound anxiety in neophyte researchers lest their research fall short of this mythological standard. The rationale for the creation of this myth may relate to bolstering researchers' egos, although why this is necessary is uncertain. Perhaps the behaviour recounted by these researchers is familiar. Ego-brushing to the point of self-aggrandisement, objectivity and maintaining a distant neutrality are stereotypically masculine characteristics, which the midwife may recognise as features of certain health care personnel (Adshead & Dickenson 1993). This stereotype has been summarised in terms of the 'outmoded macho image of invulnerability' (Martin 1993: 84), leading us to question whether, and to what extent, females, including midwives, differ. It may be that this neutral stance is not sex linked but is a coping mechanism adopted by many practitioners who function in a situation that is dominated by masculine patriarchal values and that values 'reason' and 'science' in preference to emotion and humanity.

For the researcher, the answer is also unlikely to relate simply to gender, as evidenced by Raymond Lee's important publication on researching sensitive topics (1993). The discomforts that researchers have experienced during their fieldwork have, however, been reported in detail by few. The term 'confessional tales' was coined by Van Maanen (1988: 73) to describe the embarrassments and hardships of a qualitative researcher. Juliene Lipson provides uncannily familiar examples such as, when researching a family-orientated culture, her embarrassment at failing to recognise an invitation to her family, thus causing unnecessary expense to her 'financially struggling' hosts (1989: 81). Lipson also refers to her personal reactions of frustration while working alongside 'highly educated' men in a male-dominated culture. Her inability to accept her male colleagues' dismissiveness of a woman's views brought home to her the reality of her situation compared, presumably, with the artificiality of her usual, politically correct working environment. The emotional demands of fieldwork may be manageable when interviewing because there is invariably at least one other person present to offer some form of human contact and, possibly, reassurance. Lipson reminds us that it is when the researcher is alone, undertaking the solitary tasks of transcribing and analysing the data, that painful personal doubts are likely to intrude. Similarly, the midwife's pain of caring may be delayed until the paperwork is being completed.

Despite Lipson's reassurances of its low-threat nature, the limited attention given to the vulnerability of the researcher has focused mainly on the interview. One exception, however, is the work of Gregory *et al* (1997), who pick up on Lipson's 'solitary' tasks by discussing the transcriber's role. Transcription is assumed to be emotion-free, perhaps even automatic and unconscious, but these writers suggest that rather than being immune, the transcriber is in the front line for emotional trauma. The transcriber may be more vulnerable than the researcher because, like the interviewer and those who provide care, she is in direct contact, albeit aural, with the informant rather than being insulated from painful reality by the sanitisation of the informant's words through computers and printers. The risks associated with solitary work and with direct contact with disturbing data are endorsed by an important Australian study of traumatic deaths (Driscoll *et al* 1997).

The focus on the vulnerability of the interviewer in particular is attributable to the dynamic nature of the research interview (Holland & Ramazanoglu 1994: 135). The research interview may, however, be viewed less positively. Brannen (1988: 562) suggests that psychiatrists and psychotherapists would have difficulty enduring the rigours imposed on the researcher/interviewer even though these therapists are better prepared for and protected from such experiences. She blames some of the difficulty on the length of the research interview, which is not limited to therapists' 1-hour sessions. These therapists' contacts differ from midwifery as well in that they are invariably time limited.

The time-consuming and emotionally draining nature of the interview is further endorsed by Kelly (1988: 10), who reports that the researcher may spend as much time 'chatting' with the informant as in conducting extremely long interviews. This 'chat' may offer opportunities for the informant to reconcile herself to the experience of self-disclosure (Antle May 1989) and help to 'put herself back together' after being interviewed on an emotional topic. We need also to take account of the therapeutic value of this time for the researcher, who may have similar emotional repairs to make. When undertaking interviews with relinquishing mothers and midwives, I found that that final cup of coffee with the tape recorder switched off was indescribably beneficial, even though the act of switching it off often merely moved us into a different phase of the interview. The ethical requirement for debriefing by the researcher is addressed more objectively by Alty and Rodham (1998), who recount interviewers' defensive tactics.

It might be assumed that the emotional challenge to the researcher must be less than to the informant, but Holland and Ramazanoglu (1994: 137) suggest that this may not apply. In their example, a 'gang rape' survivor had been able to undertake a 'massive amount of work on herself and the experience' before the interview, whereas the interviewer was unprepared for such horror. These researchers give as another example an interviewer who did not realise that her grieving for a parent was incomplete until an informant felt the need to unburden himself of his old grief on to her. Thus, the cathartic value of the research interview to the informant (Brannen 1988) may be at great personal cost to the interviewer. Although, ideally, the midwife has a chance to prepare herself for emotionally taxing situations, staff shortages may prevent this, as in the case study below.

The personal benefits as well as the costs become apparent in a study involving interviewing grieving mothers (Farnsworth 1996). Farnsworth explains the ways in which the reflexive approach used to interact with each of the mothers facilitated her own grieving. Farnsworth only briefly mentions the 'often painful' nature of this work (1996: 412), and the completeness of the picture is uncertain. The 'actual pain' of researching sensitive topics was identified during a study of battered women (Dunn 1991: 388). In this account, the reader senses Dunn's lack of preparation for the 'stress, deep personal involvement, role conflicts, discomfort and physical and mental effort' aggravated by 'feelings of anger and powerlessness' that this research aroused.

☐ Researchers' coping strategies and their relevance to the midwife

Having examined the extent to which the researcher/interviewer may be emotionally traumatised by direct contact during fieldwork, it is now necessary to consider the recommendations to help the researcher to cope with the potential for, or reality of, such trauma. These recommendations will lead us to contemplate their relevance to the midwife caring for the grieving mother.

The account by Dunn pleads for greater openness concerning the emotional effects of research. This contradicts the anthropologically orientated, macho, stiff-upper-lip approach (Freilich 1979; Gans 1982). Dunn advocates that researchers report '*real* observations and experiences' (1991: 390, emphasis added). She implicitly condemns mythological accounts of perfect projects and suggests that if the interviewer is prepared for a less than comfortable experience, she is likely to have her coping strategies in place sooner rather than later.

As mentioned above, emotional vulnerability in the research process focuses on the interview but may include transcription and data analysis (Lipson 1989; Dunn 1991). The focus on the interviewer is attributable to her subordinate role in the research team and poor support mechanisms (Brannen 1988), both of which are linked with her solitary role. Brannen expands on the interviewer's difficulty by describing it as 'looking in two directions at once' (1988: 563) or being pulled emotionally in the direction of both the research team and the informant. It is often assumed that the research team provides the necessary support for its emotionally vulnerable members on an informal basis. Holland and Ramazanoglu, however, indicate that, although the team may provide colleagues and opportunities for discussing emotionally disturbing and demanding interviews, this is not always possible precisely when it is needed. They conclude that 'the impact of interviews on sensitive topics on interviewers should not be under-estimated, and a support structure is advisable' (1994: 137). Brannen also recommends that safeguards should be built into the project in the form of 'researcher support', suggesting that both the data and staff morale would benefit. These safeguards were formalised in Driscoll *et al*'s large Australian study of coroners' records (1997): because the researchers were relatively isolated, a system of 'pairing' was built into the research protocol to provide peer support by ensuring the availability of an empathetic listener.

The cathartic nature of the research interview has been identified as being at personal cost to the interviewer (Lee 1981; Brannen 1988). In a light-hearted approach, Alty and Rodham (1998: 280) discuss tactics that the interviewer may use to reduce this particular 'Ouch! factor' by redirecting the conversation away from potentially painful topics. According to these authors, the interviewer soon learns such avoidance tactics, especially as such confidences may be preceded by requests to switch off the tape recorder, clearly rendering the subsequent material useless to the research. These writers' tactics, although helpful to the interviewer and to the research, would reduce the informant's benefit in the research bargain and are therefore of questionable utility in the research situation. While it may be that the midwife may inadvertently resort to such tactics as a form of self-protection, their ethical bases are dubious.

A further strategy to resolve the interviewer's emotional vulnerability (Cannon 1992) comprises the informant's increasingly active involvement in the data production. Such active involvement, through balanced rather than hierarchical input, has been suggested by feminist researchers to cope with the problems of the lack of women's voices in research (Oakley 1981; Finch 1984) but may serve a dual function. This 'collaborative' approach (Laslett & Rapoport 1975) may act to challenge the hierarchy of conventional research, which has the effect of rendering the informant passive.

Despite the recommendations mentioned above for a formalisation of researchers' support frameworks, I, like Dunn, found support in my home and from my academic colleagues as well as health professionals. Based on her personal experience, Dunn (1991: 391) makes a series of five recommendations that the researcher might utilise to reduce her emotional vulnerability. Her recommendations include an assessment of personal coping mechanisms, the activation of social support mechanisms and the sharing of experiences already alluded to. Dunn also advises that the researcher keep a daily 'log' of her thoughts, to act as a silent counsellor but possibly also eventually to contribute to the data. Her most difficult recommendation is that the researcher undertake only one interview per day; this may not be feasible if the timing of interviews is very precise, perhaps because the informant is experiencing some form of transition. The need for such support for midwives emerges in the case study below.

☐ The care of the midwife

It is clear that there are many similarities between the personal costs to the researcher and those to the midwife caring for the grieving mother. These similarities suggest that the interventions that have been recommended to assist researchers may be helpful to carers in situations of loss. I consider here whether the recommendations made in the context of research are appropriate for the midwife caring for the grieving woman.

Dunn's plea for greater openness (1991) may still be relevant for some midwives and their colleagues. In the research already mentioned, I found that the concept of professionalism still held sway with some midwives. This is what 'Bessie' told me when I asked her about sharing tears with a grieving mother:

> There are two schools of thought about it. First, there is the old school which says that you must retain your professional thing quite intact. The second view is that you grieve with the woman. I think that it really depends on the midwife and the woman. I am quite happy to hold her hand or to put my arm around her shoulder, but I think you need to stay a professional.
>
> (Mander 1994: 157)

Other health care providers have found a similar difficulty in coping with the grieving mother or couple:

It was the way [the registrar] came in several times and he just stared at us... didn't say nothing... I don't know whether he couldn't handle it.... He just stared at us. Sort of to say, 'There's nothing I can really do much'.

(Moulder 1998: 126)

That some recognition is emerging appears in a later informant's comment:

I wish there was something that you could give [the grieving mother] in the way of support. But I don't know whether that's possible really and, I don't know, perhaps the doctor isn't the right person to become involved.

(Moulder 1998: 126)

The plea for openness may relate not only to our ability to provide care, but also to our experience of providing that care. Dunn comments that 'Such pain [for the researcher] may constitute an important source of data and should be identified' (1991: 390). In the health care context, it might be suggested that experiencing the actual pain of caring for a grieving mother is part of the caring experience, and the pain of caring may help us to care more effectively. In the same way as grief provides the bereaved person with opportunities for personal growth, caring for a grieving mother may facilitate personal and professional growth and real interaction. Thus, the teaching of health care providers in general and midwives in particular needs to focus on the reality of care in loss, including teaching about genuine engagement rather than the 'rugger pass' approach.

In my research, informal support emerged as a crucial, albeit unpredictable and unreliable, phenomenon. While the coffee room or the pub after the shift ended were often mentioned, it became clear that these tended to be less helpful when all the staff were working under stress.

Although formal support structures have long been recommended for health care personnel (Cole 1993), problems exist with both the establishment and the utilisation of such services. These services are low priority in a health care system in which resources are stretched to breaking point. Similarly, in an organisation where staff may feel undervalued, the trust necessary for support services to be utilised is also lacking. Even so, Driscoll *et al*'s experience (1997) of formalising peer support for staff likely to be traumatised by their work could be relevant to health care providers. Short-term avoidance tactics (Alty & Rodham 1998) hardly seem appropriate in a caring situation.

Collaborative care, such as increasing the involvement of the mother or parents in both decision-making and the care of a baby who is dying or has died, is clearly appropriate. The benefits to the mother who 'meets' her stillborn child are well known, as is the variety of forms that this 'meeting' can take (Rådestad *et al* 1996).

The five recommendations that Dunn (1991) made in the research context are clearly applicable to midwifery care, but it may be difficult to ensure that these are put into practice in an emergency service where demands are great. Each of the midwives in my study told me of her attempts to assess a colleague's current personal coping mechanisms before allocating her to a grieving mother. Similarly, the midwife was also able to activate social support at work. The keeping of a daily log is an aspect of reflective care that many health care personnel now learn as students, but its relevance to a practising midwife is less certain. The likelihood of one midwife caring for more than one grieving mother in one spell of duty, as in the case study below, seems remote, but, as with any emergency service, such a possibility exists. A particular problem, as midwives reported, is not only with caring for the grieving mother but in making the constant emotional adjustment and readjustment when caring for mothers with very different needs (Mander 1991: 138).

■ Case study – so much to do...

The labour ward midwifery staffing level was low as a result of sickness, so it was just as well that that evening was quiet. Maureen was in charge but wasn't feeling too well. The report told me that, although there were not many women in labour, those who were with us were experiencing problems. The two women to whom I was allocated were not in labour but needed different kinds of help.

Later Maureen asked me to stay with Joanna. The report had told me that Joanna was giving birth very prematurely to a baby who could not survive, and she was finding difficulty understanding what was happening. I went into her room and introduced myself to Joanna and to Ben. Joanne had been given analgesia but was still feeling pain. The contractions were coming frequently, suggesting that the birth was imminent. Joanna's birth plan was helpful.

I realised how little I was able to do for a mother experiencing the loss of a baby. Then I rehearsed in my mind what a midwife might do to make the experience of birth more real for the mother in order to facilitate her healthy grieving. The creation of memories is crucial to our care at this time.

We talked about Joanna seeing her baby after the birth, and she and Ben thought that they would wait a few minutes before holding the baby. Joanna asked me how big the baby was likely to be; I scoured my memory for my lectures on fetal development and suggested about the size of her hand.

The minister had looked in, and both Joanna and Ben were keen for him to return after the birth; they were, however, uncertain whether they wanted the baby to be blessed or christened. They said they had chosen a name, but I avoided intruding by asking them what it was. One of my colleagues had already brought in some soft white linen ready to receive the baby. I doubted whether name bands, locks of hair or footprints would be appropriate for such a tiny being but knew that a Swedish study had shown that photographs could serve as a helpful reminder of the birth. These might or might not include the parents and might be given to them immediately, depending on how they felt.

During this waiting time, we attempted to establish a relationship by seeking shared values. We talked about the bodily feelings that Joanna would experience that would indicate that her baby was about to be born. Soon her body began to tell her that the baby was coming and he was born peacefully. Ben's tears fell on to Joanna's face as they shared their sorrow; perhaps only now were they coming to believe that their baby really could not survive. I wrapped him and Ben asked to hold him. I learned that he was to be named Kevin and wondered what unfulfilled and unfulfillable expectations this name represented. After minimal tidying and checking, I asked to be excused and left Joanna and Ben with their son.

I contacted the minister, Ian, and sought the camera. When Ian came in, he enquired how the birth had gone and how Joanna and Ben seemed. I was able to be quite positive until he asked about me. Although my contact with Joanna and Ben had made me think about all the facets of my care, I had avoided contemplating my own coping ability. I answered in terms of 'Good enough', but unconvincingly, knowing only too well that a total stranger, walking into a situation of loss, may be less than helpful.

When Kevin was suitably wrapped and lying in his miniature cradle, we prepared for his blessing. Joanna and Ben agreed that I could stay, hopefully showing my recognition of the importance of this baby. Ian's blessing of this minute person was thoughtful and we shared our tears.

Only with Ben's help was I able to make sense of the 'state-of-the-art' camera and produce photographs of this sad little family. We know that bereaved parents are sometimes dissatisfied with the photographs that are given to them, and this is likely to apply to those which I managed to produce of Joanna, Ben and Kevin.

I organised some tea for Joanna and Ben while I started work on the mountain of paperwork and computer entries. There was much duplication, but this multiplicity of checklists has been introduced in order to ensure good continuity and avoid the potentially painful repetition of questions. There were still many things to ask Joanna and Ben, and many decisions for them to make, for example concerning the post mortem, whether there would be a burial or a cremation, and whether it would be organised privately or by the Trust.

The postnatal ward midwife was unable to find Joanna a single room as there were only shared rooms free. I persisted, asking about the room for parents of stillborn babies. She interrogated me about Kevin's gestation. I persuaded her that the gestation does not affect the parents' grief, and she agreed to make the room available.

While beginning the paperwork and negotiating the room, I became aware of a woman arriving in the labour ward. Maureen interrupted my writing, asking me to see this newly arrived woman. Maureen briefly explained that the woman was about to lose her baby. I recoiled, protesting that my care and documentation were incomplete and that Joanna had yet to go to the ward. My protestations were ineffective as all the other midwives were with women who could not be left. Reluctantly, leaving Joanna's documents unfinished and being uncertain when I would ask the outstanding questions, I introduced myself to Tracy and her sister Sharon.

My questions and observations confirmed that this baby could not be born alive. Did Tracy realise this when she asked whether her baby would be OK? I explained that the outlook was not good. There had been little opportunity to get to know Tracy when, a short while later, a tiny baby girl was born. Tracy was more horrified than sorrowful. I tidied and checked, and explained to Tracy that it was all right to be sad and to cry when a baby was lost. Recalling the Swedish study, I suggested that it might be helpful for her to see her baby. She looked unconvinced and consulted Sharon. Tracy decided to see her baby, but after one quick glance her look of horror returned. I took the baby away unnamed and untouched by her mother. When I returned a midwife unknown to me was with Tracy. The night staff had arrived.

I explained to this midwife what was being done for Tracy and what was outstanding, as well as the same information with regard to Joanna and Ben. While talking to her, it dawned on me how much care Joanna and Tracy needed and how little I had been able to give. Tears of impotence began to flow, and this unknown midwife took me aside, assuring me that she would complete their care.

It was time for me to go to my warm, loving home. I learned the next day that Ben had gone home that night because neither I nor anybody else had explained that he was welcome to stay with Joanna in her double bed. Instead, both of them spent their sad and sleepless night alone.

☐ Questions

● Could the midwife manager have dealt with this situation in any other way?

● Was this midwife right to encourage Tracy to 'meet' her baby?

● How should midwives be helped to use equipment such as cameras?

● Was this midwife right to abandon Joanna and Ben in order to care for Tracy?

■ Conclusion

In the same way as perinatal loss was ignored because of health care personnel's inability to cope or deal with it, the personal costs to the researcher have been underreported. Feminist critiques of research practice and the increasing use of qualitative approaches to research, which may not be unrelated, have opened up both areas to research scrutiny, discussion and a search for coping strategies. The emotional difficulties among staff caring for parents who are bereaved are similarly inadequately discussed but may be amenable to remedy using broadly similar strategies.

■ Recommendations for clinical practice in the light of currently available evidence

1. Genuine and meaningful engagement at a fundamental level between midwives and grieving mothers and between midwife practitioners should be encouraged. The achievement of such engagement could be evaluated by the midwife in the course of her reflection on her practice, which may be assisted by a peer or supervisor.

2. It is important to establish support structures, perhaps involving reflection, that all staff may use during periods of emotional vulnerability.

3. There should be greater input by the grieving parents into their care to provide a collaborative form of care.

4. Managers need to assess coping ability before allocating a midwife to an emotionally challenging situation. This assessment may involve consultation with the midwife herself both before and after her exposure to the emotional challenge. Such issues would appropriately be addressed in the course of the midwife manager's ongoing professional development.

■ Practice check

● Are you able to recall any work situations in which you felt emotionally vulnerable?

● Do you know of any formal support systems that you might use or recommend?

● Have you ever found yourself resorting to avoidance tactics?

● Would it be helpful to you to reflect on your work in the form of a 'log'?

● Can you recall a work situation in which you were able to help a colleague who was experiencing emotional difficulty?

■ References

Adshead G, Dickenson D (1993) Why do doctors and nurses disagree? In Dickenson D, Johnson M (eds) Death, Dying and Bereavement. Open University and Sage, London, pp. 161–8.

Alty A, Rodham K (1998) The ouch! factor: problems in conducting sensitive research. Qualitative Health Research, 8(2): 275–82.

Antle May K (1989) Interview techniques in qualitative research. In Morse JM (ed.) Qualitative Nursing Research: A Contemporary Dialogue. Aspen, Rockville, pp. 188–201.

Bartos C, Mander R (1995) The implications of culture when caring for a mother following loss in pregnancy. British Journal of Midwifery, 3(11): 591–7.

Beutel M, Willner H, Deckardt R, Von Rad M, Weiner H (1996) Similarities and differences in couples' grief reactions following a miscarriage: results from a longitudinal study. Journal of Psychosomatic Research, 40(3): 245–53.

Bourne S (1968) The psychological effects of stillbirth on women and their doctors. Journal of the Royal College of General Practitioners, 16: 103–12.

Brannen J (1988) Research note: the study of sensitive subjects. Sociological Review, 36(3): 552–63.

Burnell GM, Norfleet MA (1979) Women who place their infant up for adoption: a pilot study. Patient Counselling and Health Education, (summer/fall): 169–72.

Cannon S (1992) Reflections on fieldwork in stressful settings: difficulties for the sociologist studying the treatment of breast cancer. Sociology of Health and Illness, 11: 62–77.

Chalmers I (1993) Effective care in midwifery: research, the professions and the public. Midwives Chronicle, 106(1260): 3–12.

Cochrane AL (1972) Effectiveness and efficiency. Nuffield Provincial Hospitals Trust, London.

Cole A (1993) Vital support. Nursing Times, 89(13): 16–17.

Cordell AS, Thomas N (1997) Perinatal loss: intensity and duration of emotional recovery. Omega – Journal of Death and Dying, 35(3): 297–308.

Cowles KV (1996) Cultural perspectives of grief: an expanded concept analysis. Journal of Advanced Nursing, 23(2): 287–94.

Driscoll TR, Hull BP, Mandryk JA, Mitchell RJ, Howland AS (1997) Minimizing the personal cost of involvement in research into traumatic death. Safety Science, 25: 1–3, 45–53.

Dunn L (1991) Research alert! Qualitative research may be dangerous to your health. Qualitative Health Research, 1(3): 388–92.

Dyregrov A (1991) Grief in Children: A Handbook for Adults. Kingsley, London.

Farnsworth EB (1996) Reflexivity and qualitative family research: insider's perspectives in bereaving the loss of a child. Marriage and Family Review, 24: 3–4, 399–415.

Finch J (1984) 'It's great to have someone to talk to': the ethics and politics of interviewing women . In Bell C, Roberts H (eds) Social Researching: Politics Problems and Practice. Routledge & Kegan Paul, London, pp. 70–87.

Forrest G, Standish E, Baum J (1982) Support after perinatal death: a study of support and counselling after perinatal bereavement. British Medical Journal, 285: 1475–79.

Freilich M (1979) Fieldwork: an introduction. In Freilich M (ed) Marginal Natives: Anthropologists at Work. Harper & Row, New York, pp. 1–38.

Frost M, Condon JT (1996) The psychological sequelae of miscarriage: a critical review of the literature. Australian and New Zealand Journal of Psychiatry, 30(1): 54–62.

Gans HJ (1982) The participant observer as a human being: observations on the personal aspects of fieldwork. In Burgess RG (ed.) Field Research: A Sourcebook and Field Manual. George Allen & Unwin, London, pp. 53–61.

Gohlish M (1985) Stillbirth. Midwife, Health Visitor and Community Nurse, 21(1): 16.

Gregory D, Russell CK, Phillips LR (1997) Beyond textual perfection: transcribers as vulnerable persons. Qualitative Health Research, 7(2): 294–300.

Gribbin J (1998) Review: How not to do it. New Scientist, 157(2116): 41.

Holland J, Ramazanoglu C (1994) Power and interpretation in researching young women's sexuality. In Maynard M, Purvis J (eds) Researching women's lives from a feminist perspective. Taylor & Francis, London, pp. 125–48.

Hunfeld JA, Mourik MM, Passchier J, Tibboel D (1996) Do couples grieve differently following infant loss? Psychological Reports, 79(2): 407–10

Hunfeld JA, Wladimiroff JW, Passchier J (1997) Prediction and course of grief four years after perinatal loss due to congenital anomalies: a follow-up study. British Journal of Medical Psychology, 70(1): 85–91.

Iles S (1989) The loss of early pregnancy. In Oates MR (ed) Psychological Aspects of Obstetrics and Gynaecology. Baillière Tindall, London, pp. 126–38.

Jacob SR (1993) An analysis of the concept of grief. Journal of Advanced Nursing, 18: 1787–94.

Johnson MP, Puddifoot JE (1996) The grief response in the partners of women who miscarry. British Journal of Medical Sociology, 69: 14, 313–27.

Kalish RA (1985) Death, Grief and Caring Relationships, 2nd edn. Brooks Cole, California.

Kelly L (1988) Surviving sexual violence. Polity Press, Cambridge.

Kübler-Ross E (1970) On Death and Dying. Tavistock Publications, London.

Laslett B, Rapoport R (1975) Collaborative interviewing and interactive research. Journal of Marriage and the Family, 37: 968–77.

Lee C, Slade P (1996) Miscarriage as a traumatic event: a review of the literature and new implications for intervention. Journal of Psychosomatic Research, 40(3): 235–44.

Lee RM (1981) Interreligious courtship and marriage in Northern Ireland. PhD thesis, University of Edinburgh.

Lee RM (1993) Doing Research on Sensitive Topics. Sage, London.

Leon IG (1990) When a Baby Dies: Psychotherapy for Pregnancy and Newborn Loss. Yale University Press, Yale.

Lilford R, Stratton P, Godsil S, Prasad A (1994) A randomised trial of routine versus selective counselling in perinatal bereavement from congenital disease. British Journal of Obstetrics and Gynaecology, 101(4): 291–6.

Lin SX, Lasker JN (1996) Patterns of grief reaction after pregnancy loss. American Journal of Orthopsychiatry, 66(2): 262–71.

Lindemann E (1944) Symptomatology and management of acute grief. American Journal of Psychiatry, 101: 141–9.

Lipson JG (1989) The use of self in ethnographic research. In Morse JM (ed.) Qualitative Nursing Research: A Contemporary Dialogue. Aspen, Rockville, pp. 73–89.

Lumley J (1980) The image of the fetus in the first trimester. Birth, 7(1): 5–12.

Mander R (1991) Midwifery care of the grieving mother – how the decisions are made. Midwifery, 7(3): 133–42.

Mander R (1994) Loss and Bereavement in Childbearing. Blackwell Scientific, Oxford.

Mander R (1995) The Care of the Mother Grieving a Baby Relinquished for Adoption. Avebury, Aldershot.

Martin J (1993) Doctor's mask on pain. In Dickenson D, Johnson M (eds) Death, Dying and Bereavement. Open University/Sage, London, pp. 83–4.

Moulder C (1998) Understanding Pregnancy Loss: Perspectives and Issues in Care. Macmillan, London.

Neugebauer R, Kline J, Shrout P *et al* (1997) Major depressive disorder in the six months after miscarriage. Journal of the American Medical Association, 277(5): 383–8.

Nolan ML, Hicks C (1997) Aims, processes and problems of antenatal education as identified by three groups of childbirth teachers. Midwifery, 13(4): 179–88.

Oakley A (1981) Interviewing women: a contradiction in terms. In Roberts H (ed.) Doing Feminist Research. Routledge, London, pp. 30–61.

Parkes CM (1972) Bereavement. International Universities Press, New York.

Pine VR, Brauer C (1986) Parental grief: a synthesis of theory research and intervention. In Rando TA (ed.) Parental Loss of Child. Research Press, Champaign IL.

Prendiville W, O'Kelly F, Allwright S, Mcguinness N (1997) The management of first trimester miscarriage by general practitioners in Ireland. Irish Journal of Medical Science, 166(1): 3–6.

Rådestad I, Nordin C, Steineck G, Sjogren B (1996) Stillbirth is no longer managed as a non-event: a nationwide study in Sweden. Birth, 23(4): 209–16.

Rajan L (1994) Social isolation and support in pregnancy loss. Health Visitor, 67(3): 97–101.

Rees C (1997) An Introduction to Research for Midwives. Hochland & Hochland, Hale.

Robinson DS, McKenna HP (1998) Loss: an analysis of a concept of particular interest to nursing. Journal of Advanced Nursing, 27(4): 779–84.

Rynearson EK (1987) Psychotherapy of pathologic grief: revisions and limitations. Psychiatric Clinics of North America, 10(3): 487–99.

Salvesen KA, Oyen L, Schmidt N, Malt UF, Elk-Nes SH (1997) Comparison of long term psychological responses of women after pregnancy termination due to fetal anomalies and after perinatal loss. Ultrasound in Obstetrics and Gynaecology, 9(2): 80–5.

Schaap AHP, Wolf H, Bruinse HW, Barkhofvandelande S, Treffers PE (1997) Long-term impact of perinatal bereavement – comparison of grief reactions after intrauterine versus neonatal death. European Journal of Obstetrics, Gynaecology and Reproductive Biology, 75(2): 161–7.

Stroebe W, Stroebe MS (1987) Bereavement and Health: The Psychological and Physical Consequences of Partner Loss. Cambridge University Press, Cambridge.

Thomas V, Striegel P (1995) Stress and grief of a perinatal loss – integrating qualitative and quantitative methods. Omega – Journal of Death and Dying, 30(4): 299–311.

Van Maanen J (1988) Tales of the Field. University of Chicago Press, Chicago.

Worth NJ (1997) Becoming a father to a stillborn child. Clinical Nursing Research, 6(1): 71–89.

■ Suggested further reading

Mander R (1994) Loss and Bereavement in Childbearing. Blackwell Scientific, Oxford.

Shaffir WB, Stebbins RA (eds) (1991) Experiencing Fieldwork: An inside view of qualitative research. Sage, London.

Chapter 4

From pregnancy to lactation: changing relations between mother and baby – a biological perspective

Mary McNabb and Suzanne Colson

■ Introduction

From a biological perspective, the nutritional and developmental needs of the embryo, fetus and infant are met by a series of reciprocal interactions between mother and offspring that extend from conception to spontaneous weaning. These successive events are regulated by neurohormonal and enzymatic changes that demonstrate continuity and discontinuity, from pregnancy and parturition, to lactation and suckling. This chapter will identify particular examples of continuity and discontinuity, with a view to highlighting the dynamics of maternal–fetal–neonatal interactions from pregnancy to spontaneous weaning.

☐ The oxytocin experience

Oxytocin, in both mother and baby, provides one of the clearest examples of continuity. Released centrally and peripherally during and after pregnancy, oxytocin has been implicated in a wide variety of physiological events, including sexual activity, myometrial and myoepithelial contractions, prolactin stimulation and inhibition, glucose metabolism, long-term weight gain and aspects of infant and maternal behaviour (Newton & Newton 1967; Samson *et al* 1986; Fuchs & Fuchs 1991; Parker *et al* 1991; Widmaier 1991; McCarthy *et al* 1992; Herbert 1994; Wakerley *et al* 1994; Breton *et al* 1995; Da Costa *et al* 1996; Neumann *et al* 1996; Yuan & Pan 1996; Douglas *et al* 1998; Mitchell *et al* 1998; Russell & Leng 1998; Uvnas-Moberg *et al* 1998).

Experimental evidence from rats suggests that the distinct and highly dynamic expression of oxytocin in maternal brain cells during pregnancy and lactation is regulated by changing levels of oestrogen and progesterone, both before and after birth (Jirikowski 1992; Broad *et al* 1993; Crowley *et al* 1995; Thomas *et al* 1995; Jiang and Wakerley 1997). Uterine receptors for oxytocin increase in number from early pregnancy, while those in the mammary gland begin to increase just before parturition, rising more rapidly at the onset of lactation and disappearing during weaning (Fuchs & Fuchs 1991; Wakerley *et al* 1994; Leung *et al* 1998). Although the contribution made by fetal oxytocin to myometrial contraction remains uncertain, recent findings on the release of neonatal oxytocin in response to stroking, touch and warm temperature have demonstrated its capacity to stimulate a number of neurohormonal and metabolic changes that promote long-term weight gain (Dawood *et al* 1978a, 1978b; Uvnas-Moberg *et al* 1993, 1998; Mueller-Heubach *et al* 1995; Bjorkstrand *et al* 1996).

Current evidence on humans suggests that peripheral concentrations of oxytocin in the maternal circulation are significantly lower during labour than they are during suckling. In samples taken at 1-minute intervals before and during labour at term, the frequency of oxytocin pulses increased significantly during labour, although mean peak plasma values remained around $1.0 \, \mu U/ml$ and most of the higher values were obtained just around birth (Fuchs *et al* 1991). In women fully suckling their babies, peripheral concentrations of oxytocin obtained during feeding were found to increase from $4.6 \, \mu U/ml$ at 2–4 weeks postpartum, to $8.6 \, \mu U/ml$ at 15–24 weeks (Johnston & Amico 1986). These findings may be explained by other evidence suggesting that oxytocin release during labour and birth may facilitate a more pulsatile pattern of oxytocin release during suckling. In a recent study comparing oxytocin pulses during suckling on the second day following birth, women who gave birth vaginally had significantly more oxytocin pulses during the first 10 minutes of suckling compared with those who had an emergency caesarean section (Nissen *et al* 1996).

Other examples of continuity are evident in the reduction of maternal energy expenditure that characterises pregnancy and lactation, the increased rate of intestinal iron and calcium absorption that is common to the second half of pregnancy and lactation, and the maternal capacity to regulate both fetal and neonatal temperature (Illingsworth *et al* 1986; Acolet *et al* 1989; Uvnas-Moberg 1989; Uvnas-Moberg and Winberg 1989; Ludington-Hoe *et al* 1991; Christensson *et al* 1998; Zhu *et al* 1998).

☐ **Distinct characteristics of fetal and neonatal metabolism**

On the other hand, in a key area such as glucose homeostasis, evidence of discontinuity is much more apparent, as this regulatory activity is abruptly transferred from the mother to the neonate at the moment of birth. Throughout pregnancy, the fetus is continually supplied through the placenta with a diet rich in carbohydrates and amino acids but relatively low in lipids. In addition to the essential fatty acids that support growth and brain development, supplies of non-essential lipids are stored in fetal adipose tissue and the liver, particularly during the latter half of pregnancy. Although lipids become an important substrate for energy metabolism during early postnatal life, unlike glucose, lactate, alanine and ketones, they are not readily used as a source of energy during fetal life (Bougnères *et al* 1986; Atkins & Clandinin 1990; Herrera *et al* 1992).

When the continuous supply of maternal glucose is suddenly terminated with the cessation of the placental circulation very soon after birth, the newborn moves to intermittent supplies of a liquid substance – milk – that is rich in medium- and long-chain fatty acids but low in carbohydrate. Immediately following birth, carbohydrate is no longer ingested as glucose but as lactose, a disaccharide that needs to be hydrolysed in order to release equal amounts of galactose and glucose (Kliegman & Sparks 1985; Sparks 1992). At the same time, previously high levels of insulin suddenly fall and remain relatively unresponsive for several days. In vitro evidence suggests that, following birth, insulin secretion does not seem to respond particularly effectively to the usual physiological stimuli (Sperling *et al* 1974). This may be because of the inhibitory effect of adrenaline on insulin release, and the extensive remodelling and reduced growth of the endocrine pancreas, including the beta cell population, that occurs immediately after birth (Atkins & Clandinin 1990; Scaglia *et al* 1997; Petrik *et al* 1998). This sequence of events seems to suggest that birth is accompanied by a sudden and dramatic metabolic switch from carbohydrate to fat metabolism that could easily endanger glucose homeostasis in the neonate, particularly during the first 3 days of extrauterine life (Widmaier 1990; Cowett *et al* 1997).

The remainder of this chapter will explore changes in maternal and fetal metabolism during the second half of pregnancy and labour that seem to prepare both mother and offspring for the transition from placental to mammary nutrition. Current experimental evidence suggests that, during the period of suckling, glucose homeostasis is less tightly regulated than after weaning, when the infant returns, physiologically speaking, to a high-carbohydrate diet (Issad *et al* 1990; Widmaier 1990; Girard *et al* 1992; Macho *et al* 1995; Gardner *et al* 1997; Cowett *et al* 1998).

■ It is assumed that you are already aware of the following:

● Glycogenesis – the pathway by which glucose is converted in successive stages to glycogen;

● Gluconeogenesis – the pathway by which glucose is synthesised from non-carbohydrate sources, notably lactate, pyruvate and glycerol;

● Lipogenesis – the pathway by which triglycerol is synthesised from fatty acids and glycerol;

- Lipolysis – the pathways by which stored fat is broken down into glycerol and fatty acids;

- Ketogenesis – the pathway by which fatty acids are converted in the liver to ketone bodies.

■ Effect of maternal catabolism to facilitate fetal anabolism during the latter half of pregnancy

Research findings on well-nourished women indicate that maternal metabolism tends to shift from avid anabolism to prolific catabolism during the second half of pregnancy. In the first half of pregnancy, increased insulin secretion and a heightened sensitivity to insulin facilitates an increased conversion of glucose into adipose tissue fatty acids and enhances the uptake of all nutrients by maternal tissues (Fraser 1991; Brelje *et al* 1993; Sorenson *et al* 1993). During this period, the accumulation of maternal adipose tissue and increased blood volume are the main components of the weight gain.

By around 28 weeks' gestation, metabolism shows an accelerated tendency towards catabolism, and weight gain for the remainder of pregnancy is primarily from the growing fetus and placenta. Maternal fat stores accumulated during the first half of pregnancy are readily hydrolysed in preference to glucose in order to meet maternal energy requirements. This tendency is particularly evident following an overnight fast. Compared with the non-pregnant state, fasting plasma glucose and amino acid concentrations are significantly lower, while those of free fatty acids, cholesterol and ketone are significantly higher, during the third trimester (Paterson *et al* 1967; Felig & Lynch 1970; Metzinger *et al* 1982). To facilitate the diversion of nutrients away from maternal organs during the latter half of pregnancy, there is a marked degree of insulin resistance and glucose intolerance, particularly in adipose tissue (Herrera *et al* 1990; Caruso *et al* 1998). In response to a 50 g glucose load during the latter half of pregnancy, plasma glucose levels rise over a longer time period, peak values and those at 2 hours being higher than in early pregnancy despite a significant rise in insulin secretion (Fraser 1991).

In terms of circulating nutrients, these changes result in a more prolonged hyperglycaemia in the fed maternal state, followed by rapid lipolysis and ketogenesis in the fasted state. This produces *lower* maternal fasting glucose levels than in the first half of pregnancy and *higher* levels of free fatty acids and ketones. In terms of fetal nutrition, these maternal changes mean higher and more prolonged periods of hyperglycaemia followed by *increased* supplies of free fatty acids and ketones. Since the placenta and mammary glands are excluded from this state of insulin resistance, these organs utilise the increased vascular concentrations of glucose, lipids and ketones to meet both the present and future needs of the offspring (Herrera *et al* 1988; Lopez-Luna *et al* 1994).

■ Fetal metabolism during the latter half of pregnancy

In direct contrast to that of the mother, fetal metabolism during the second half of pregnancy is characterised by an avid state of anabolism marked by a fourfold increase in weight between 26 and 40 weeks gestation. From 26 to 30 weeks, non-fat and fat calories contribute equally to the energy content of the body. Beyond that point, however, fat accumulation increasingly predominates, and by the end of pregnancy the *deposition of fat* accounts for over 90 per cent of the calories accumulated by the human fetus (Feldman *et al* 1992). Maternally derived glucose provides the main precursor for lipid synthesis and the accumulation of hepatic glycogen stores. Glycogen is stored in fetal tissues from as early as 9 weeks' gestation and increases significantly during the third trimester (Blackburn & Loper 1992; Philipps 1992). While the largest store of glycogen is found in the liver, glycogen is also, after 24 weeks gestation, stored in skeletal and cardiac muscle. By term, the well-nourished fetus has 2–3 times more glycogen in skeletal muscle and 10 times more in cardiac muscle than the adult (Page *et al* 1981).

Current evidence from animal and human studies suggests that the increased placental transport of essential and non-essential lipids during the latter half of pregnancy is used to synthesise triglycerides for adipose tissue stores and phospholipids for a variety of plasma membranes, as well as to accumulate very long chain fatty acids for rapid growth in the neural, retinal and lung tissues, particularly during the latter half of pregnancy (Coleman 1989; Carlson 1992; Herrera *et al* 1992; Stephenson *et al* 1993). At the same time, the complete permeability of the placenta to ketone bodies provides the fetus with an additional substrate that may be used as an energetic fuel and for lipogenesis (Seccombe *et al* 1977; Schambaugh 1985; Bougnères *et al* 1986; Harding and Evans 1991). The concentration of ketone bodies in the human maternal circulation increases during the third trimester, and positive correlations have been found between maternal and fetal concentrations, with a concentration gradient from mother to fetus (Paterson *et al* 1967; Sabata *et al* 1968). Current experimental evidence suggests that while the fetus has a very low capacity for ketogenesis, a number of fetal tissues, notably the brain, heart, liver, kidneys and brown adipose tissues, have been shown to possess the enzymes required to utilise ketone bodies, and their activity has been shown to increase during periods of maternal fasting or when the mother is fed a high-fat diet (Dahlquist *et al* 1972; Girard 1975; Herrera *et al* 1992).

The capacity of the rapidly growing brain to utilise ketones seems to increase from late fetal to neonatal life. In experimental studies on rats following birth, transport systems for the uptake of ketones in the brain have been shown to operate more efficiently than those for glucose (Nehlig & De Vasconcelos 1993). This enhanced capacity of the neonatal brain to utilise ketones coincides with the sharp increase in dietary lipids at the onset of suckling, which provide the liver with the necessary substrate for ketogenesis (Williams 1992). Current findings on human infants suggest that the capacity of the fetal liver to convert fatty acids to ketones matures during the last 10 weeks of gestation (de Boissieu *et al* 1995).

■ The endocrine pancreas in fetal and neonatal life

The opposing hormones insulin and glucagon behave very differently during fetal and neonatal life. By mid-gestation, the fetal pancreas is functionally responsive to variations in glucose level, and there is generally a positive relationship between maternal and fetal glucose concentrations and circulating levels of fetal insulin. During fetal life, glucose seems to regulate specific growth-promoting aspects of insulin (Hole *et al* 1988; Oliver *et al* 1993; Carver *et al* 1996; Bergsten *et al* 1998). Receptors for insulin have been identified in a number of tissues by mid-gestation, their number and affinity appearing to increase towards term, when they are significantly more numerous than is found in corresponding adult tissue (Ktorza *et al* 1985; Menon & Sperling 1988; Fowden 1989). Insulin plays a dominant role in promoting fetal anabolism during the second half of pregnancy. In a variety of experimental studies (Simmons *et al* 1978; Granner *et al* 1983; Chaffin *et al* 1995; M'Zali *et al* 1997), insulin has been found to:

- enhance maternal–fetal glucose transfer and fetal glucose uptake and utilisation;

- promote the accretion of protein;

- increase cell size and cell proliferation;

- stimulate the hepatic synthesis of glycogen and lipids;

- *inhibit* the rate-limiting enzyme for gluconeogenesis – the synthesis of glucose from non-carbohydrate sources.

While the endocrine pancreas has the capacity to secrete glucagon during fetal life, its characteristic metabolic actions do not seem to function very effectively in utero. In contrast to those for insulin, hepatic receptors for glucagon are low in number and do not seem to be connected to their intracellular pathways. Current in vitro findings from human studies suggest an increased hepatic activity of enzymes regulating gluconeogenesis during the last trimester, and experiments on lambs indicate that, in late gestation, the fetus demonstrates the capacity for gluconeogenesis during *prolonged* maternal fasting. However, in contrast to the situation in the adult, reduced plasma insulin rather than increased glucagon seems to mediate this response (Ktorza *et al* 1985; Dalinghaus *et al* 1991; Sadava *et al* 1992). Taken together, these findings strongly indicate that while the enzymatic capacity for endogenous glucose production is established during the last trimester, in contrast to the adult, it is not stimulated by glucagon.

■ Labour and birth

Recent findings suggest that maternal requirements for glucose may be *reduced* during labour. Like all smooth muscle, the myometrium has been shown to have a low energy requirement and an increased capacity for glycogen storage. Myometrial glycogen stores increase up to 10-fold during pregnancy and are used as a predominant source of energy for myometrial contractions during and after labour (Wedenberg *et al* 1990; Steingrims-dottir *et al* 1993). At the same time, skeletal muscle activity is reduced, and it has been suggested that maternal neocortical or higher brain requirements for glucose may also decline during labour as women become remote from the verbal communications around them (Odent 1992, 1994). On the fetal side, the increased transplacental supply of ketones during labour coincides with a 10-fold rise in catecholamine level between early labour and birth. In conjunction with the changes in environmental conditions, this surge in noradrenaline and adrenaline seems to be the single most important factor regulating the shift from glucose to lipid metabolism and from intrauterine to extrauterine life (Bistoletti *et al* 1983; Bahnsen *et al* 1984; Lagercrantz & Slotkin 1986; Lagercrantz & Marcus 1992).

■ From placental to mammary nutrition

Following birth, glucagon levels in the infant rise 3–5-fold, while insulin concentrations fall or remain at a very low range of concentrations during the early neonatal period. Experimental findings suggest that this dramatic fall in the insulin-to-glucagon ratio is stimulated almost exclusively by the earlier rise in catecholamine level (Girard *et al* 1992; Sperling 1994). In the newborn, high concentrations of adrenaline and glucagon, along with *low* concentrations of insulin, provide a powerful stimulus to mobilise glycogen and triglycerides from a variety of tissues, including liver, muscle and adipose tissue stores, all of which are abundant in well-nourished human infants at term (Christensson *et al* 1992; Nedergaard & Cannon 1992; Symonds *et al* 1995).

At the same time, the neonate uses the adrenaline surge and maturation of thyroid hormone activity to produce heat from the lipolysis of brown adipose tissue, which constitutes 1.4 per cent of body weight in newborn humans (Fisher & Polk 1994). In relation to thermogenesis, human infants following birth are categorised as having a low or moderate capacity for non-shivering thermogenesis. In this biological category, 'mothers protect their offspring by arranging a nest and by using their own body as a source of heat' (Christensson *et al* 1992: 488).

When physical contact between mother and infant is maintained following birth, peripheral concentrations of oxytocin in the maternal circulation seem to be higher in the first hour than immediately before birth (Nissen *et al* 1995). At the same time, the neonate appears to be guided to the breast by smell (Varendi *et al* 1994). During the first days of extrauterine life, the newborn demonstrates a few instinctive actions for finding and latching on to the new source of nourishment. Biologically, it is the suckling baby who takes the initiative in breastfeeding (Pryor 1963). The wrapping-around effect of the characteristically flexed body in contact with the physical contours of the mother's body seems to trigger these reflexes, while the infant's cues elicit maternal responses in a reciprocal fashion (Uvnas-Moberg 1996; Uvnas-Moberg *et al* 1998). Under physiological conditions, maternal and neonatal oxytocin is released simultaneously, stimulating metabolic and behavioural effects that promote further maternal–neonatal contact.

In the first few hours after birth, high circulating levels of catecholamines, glucagon and thyroxine stimulate glycolysis and lipolysis in the neonate. In this way, glycogen stores are broken down to glucose, and stored fats are broken down to fatty acids and glycerol. In the liver, newly released fatty acids together with those absorbed from the gut following suckling are used to form ketone bodies, while endogenous glycerol, lactate and galactose from colostrum are used to synthesise glucose. Although catecholamines in the neonate begin to decline around 30 minutes following birth, glucagon levels remain elevated and, in the rat model, the entire suckling period is characterised by high plasma glucagon and low plasma insulin level (Lagercrantz & Slotkin 1986; Girard *et al* 1992).

High concentrations of glucagon in the neonate seem to regulate the expression of two hepatic enzymes – pyruvate kinase and phosphoenolypyruvate carboxykinase – involved in glycolysis and gluconeogenesis. In experimental studies on newborn rats, glucagon has been shown to inhibit the expression of the former and stimulate the latter (Lyonnet *et al* 1988). This finding suggests that, following the utilisation of glycogen stores in the first 12–24 hours after birth, glucagon inhibits glycolysis and stimulates the increased production of glucose from non-carbohydrate sources. The replenishment of hepatic glycogen stores does not seem to be a feature of neonatal metabolism (Girard *et al* 1992).

This metabolic switch from glucose to lipid metabolism seems to be *inhibited* by hyperglycaemia. In experimental studies on newborn rats, glucose infusion inhibits glycogenolysis and, in a recent study on humans, elevated umbilical cord glucose levels were highly predictive of delayed lactogenesis (Martin *et al* 1981; Chen *et al* 1998). These findings suggest that elevated glucose values following birth may also inhibit the infant's desire for suckling.

Experimental findings from rats have demonstrated that, in contrast to the adult, the neonate does not mount a neuroendocrine stress response to glucoprivation (Widmaier 1990). This finding has been confirmed in a noninvasive experiment on appropriately grown infants at 35 and 40 weeks' gestation. During the first week of life, blood glucose concentrations ranging from 1.38 to 6.68 mmol/l showed no correlation with the functional status of the brainstem (Hawdon *et al* 1992; Cowett *et al* 1997).

■ Recommendations for clinical practice in the light of currently available evidence

1. Taken together, these research findings challenge current hospital practices which tend to *separate* mother and infant repeatedly during the first hours following birth. Removing the afterbirth, carrying out routine observations, monitoring and treating 'neonatal hypoglycaemia' and a lack of facilities for bed-sharing may all interfere with neurohormonal and metabolic changes that depend on physical contact between the mother and neonate (Girard *et al* 1992; Lau *et al* 1992; Nissen *et al* 1996; McKenna *et al* 1997; Smith *et al* 1997; van Oers *et al* 1998).

2. In biological terms, the period of suckling seems to 'direct' the neonatal pancreas to follow a particular pattern of development that appears to conclude at spontaneous weaning. Practices that interfere with this critical period may have negative implications for health in later life (Issad *et al* 1990; Macho *et al* 1995; Ladd *et al* 1996; Gardner *et al* 1997; Sarvetnick 1997).

■ Practice check

● Do you promote undisturbed physical contact between mother and baby as a key priority during the first couple of hours following birth?

● What research evidence on neonatal glucose metabolism currently informs early neonatal care in your unit?

● What research evidence is currently used to support screening for 'neonatal hypoglycaemia' in your unit?

■ References

Acolet D, Sleath K, Whitelaw A (1989) Oxygenation, heart rate and temperature in very low birth weight infants during skin-to-skin contact with their mothers. Acta Paediatrica Scandinavica, 78: 189–93.

Atkins J, Clandinin MT (1990) Nutritional significance of factors affecting carnitine dependent transport of fatty acids in neonates: a review. Nutrition Research, 10: 117–28.

Bahnsen M, Burrin JM, Johnston DG, Pernet A, Walker M, Alberti GMM (1984) Mechanisms of catecholamine effects on ketogenesis. American Journal of Physiology, 247: 173–80.

Bergsten P, Aoyagi K, Persson E, Eriksson UJ, Hellerstrom C (1998) Appearance of glucose-induced insulin release in fetal rat B-cells. Journal of Endocrinology, 158: 115–20.

Bistoletti P, Nylund L, Largercrantz H, Hjemdahl P, Strom H (1983) Fetal scalp catecholamines during labour. American Journal of Obstetrics and Gynecology, 147(7): 785–8.

Bjorkstrand E, Eriksson M, Uvnas-Moberg K (1996) Evidence of a peripheral and a central effect of oxytocin on pancreatic hormone release in rats. Neuroendocrinology, 63: 377–83.

Blackburn ST, Loper DL (1992) Maternal Fetal and Neonatal Physiology: A Clinical Perspective. WB Saunders, Philadelphia.

Boissieu D de, Rocchiccioli F, Kalack N, Bougnères PF (1995) Ketone body turnover at term and in premature newborns in the first 2 weeks after birth. Biology of the Neonate, 67: 84–93.

Bougnères PF, Lemmel C, Ferre P, Bier DM (1986) Ketone body transport in the neonate and infant. Journal of Clinical Investigation, 177: 42–8.

Brelje T Clarke, Scharp DW, Lacy PE et al (1993) Effect of homologous placental lactogens, prolactins, and growth hormones on islet B-cell division and insulin secretion in rat, mouse, and human islets: implications for placental lactogen regulation of islet function during pregnancy. Endocrinology, 132(2): 879–87.

Breton C, Pechoux C, Morel G, Zingg HH (1995) Oxytocin receptor messenger ribonucleic acid: characterization, regulation, and cellular localization in the rat pituitary gland. Endocrinology, 136(7): 2928–36.

Broad KD, Kendrick KM, Sirinathsingji DJS, Keverne EB (1993) Changes in oxytocin immunoreactivity and mRNA expression in the sheep brain during pregnancy, parturition and lactation and in response to oestrogen and progesterone. Journal of Neuroendocrinology, 5: 435–44.

Carlson SE (1992) Very long chain fatty acids in the developing retina and brain. In Polin RA and Fox WW (eds) Fetal and Neonatal Physiology. WB Saunders, Philadelphia, pp. 341–5.

Caruso A, Paradisi G, Ferrazani S et al (1998) Effect of maternal carbohydrate metabolism on fetal growth. Obstetrics and Gynaecology, 192(1): 8–12.

Carver TD, Anderson SM, Aldoretta PW, Hay W (1996) Effect of low-level basal plus marked 'pulsatile' hyperglycaemia on insulin secretion in fetal sheep. American Journal of Physiology, 271: E865–71.

Chaffin DG, Clark RM, McCracken D, Phillips AF (1995) Effect of hypoinsulinemia on growth in the fetal rabbit. Biology of the Neonate, 67: 186–93.

Chen DC, Nommsen-Rivers L, Dewey KG, Lonnerdal B (1998) Stress during labor and delivery and early lactation performance. American Journal of Clinical Nutrition, 68: 335–44.

Christensson K, Siles C, Moreno L et al (1992) Temperature, metabolic adaptation and crying in healthy full-term newborns cared for skin-to-skin or in a cot. Acta Paediatrica, 81: 488–93.

Christensson K, Bhat GJ, Amadi BC, Eriksson B, Hojer B (1998) Randomised study of skin-to-skin versus incubator care for rewarming low-risk hypothermic neonates. Lancet, 352: 1115.

Coleman RA (1989) The role of the placenta in lipid metabolism and transport. Seminars in Perinatology, 13(3): 180–91.

Cowett RM, Howard GM, Johnson J, Vohr B (1997) Brain stem auditory-evoked response in relation to neonatal glucose metabolism. Biology of the Neonate, 71: 31–6.

Cowett RM, Rapoza RE, Gelardi NL (1998) The contribution of glucose to neonatal glucose homeostasis in the lamb. Metabolism, 47(10): 1239–44.

Crowley RS, Insel TR, O'Keefe JA (1995) Increased accumulation of oxytocin messenger ribonucleic acid in the hypothalamus of the female rat: induction by long term estradiol and progesterone administration and subsequent progesterone withdrawal. Endocrinology, 136(1): 224–31.

Da Costa APC, Guevara-Guzman RG, Ohkura S, Goode JA, Kendrick KM (1996) The role of oxytocin release in the paraventricular nucleus in the control of maternal behaviour in the sheep. Journal of Neuroendocrinology, 8: 163–77.

Dahlquist G, Persson U, Persson B (1972) The activity of D–B-hydroxybutyrate dehydrogenase in fetal, infant and adult rat brain and the influence of starvation. Biology of the Neonate, 20: 40–50.

Dalinghaus M, Rudolph CD, Rudolph AM (1991) Effects of maternal fasting on hepatic gluconeogenesis and glucose metabolism in fetal lambs. Journal of Developmental Physiology, 16: 267–75.

Dawood MY, Raghavan KS, Pociask C, Fuchs F (1978a) Oxytocin in human pregnancy and parturition. Obstetrics and Gynaecology, 51(2): 138–43.

Dawood MY, Wang CF, Gupta R, Fuchs F (1978b) Fetal contribution to oxytocin in human labour. Obstetrics and Gynaecology, 52(2): 205–9.

Douglas AJ, Johnstone HA, Wigger A, Landgraf R, Russell JA, Neumann ID (1998) The role of endogenous opioids in neurohypophysial and hypothalamo-pituitary-adrenal axis hormone secretory responses to stress in pregnant rats. Journal of Endocrinology, 158: 285–93.

Feldman M, Van Aerde JE, Clandinin MT (1992) Lipid accretion in the fetus and newborn. In Polin RA, Fox WW (eds) Fetal and Neonatal Physiology. WB Saunders, Philadelphia, pp. 299–314.

Felig P, Lynch V (1970) Starvation in human pregnancy: hypoglycemia, hypoinsulinemia, and hyperketonemia. Science, 170: 9902.

Fisher DA, Polk DH (1994) The ontogenesis of thyroid function and actions. In Tulchinsky D, Little AB (eds) Maternal and Fetal Endocrinology. WB Saunders, Philadelphia, pp. 322–33.

Fowden AL (1989) The role of insulin in prenatal growth. Journal of Developmental Physiology, 12:173–82.

Fraser RB (1991) Carbohydrate metabolism. In Hytten F, Chamberlain G (eds) Clinical Physiology in Obstetrics. Blackwell Scientific, Oxford, pp. 204–12.

Fuchs A-R, Fuchs F (1991) Physiology of parturition. In Gabbe SG, Niebyl JR, Simpson JL (eds) Obstetrics, Normal and Problem Pregnancies. Churchill Livingstone, New York, pp. 147–74.

Fuchs A-R, Romero R, Keefe D, Parra M, Oyarzun E, Behnke E (1991) Oxytocin secretion and human parturition: pulse frequency and duration increase during spontaneous labor. American Journal of Obstetrics and Gynecology, 165(5): 1515–23.

Gardner SG, Bingley PJ, Sawtell Weeks S, Gale EAM (1997) Rising incidence of insulin dependent diabetes in children aged under 5 years in the Oxford region: time trend analysis. British Medical Journal, 315: 713–17.

Girard GR (1975) Metabolic fuels of the fetus. Israeli Journal of Medical Science, 11(6): 591–600.

Girard J, Ferre P, Pegorier J-P, Duee P-H (1992) Adaptations of glucose and fatty acid metabolism during perinatal period and suckling–weaning transition. Physiological Reviews, 172(2): 507–62.

Granner D, Andreone T, Sabaki K, Beale EG (1983) Inhibition of transcription of the phosphenol pyruvate carboxykinase gene by insulin. Nature, 305: 549–51.

Harding JE, Evans PC (1991) B-hydroxybutyrate is an alternative substrate for the fetal sheep brain. Journal of Developmental Physiology, 16: 2939.

Hawdon JM, Ward Platt MP, Aynsley-Green A (1992) Patterns of metabolic adaptation for preterm and term infants in the first neonatal week. Archives of Diseases in Childhood, 67: 57–65.

Herbert J (1994) Oxytocin and sexual behaviour. British Medical Journal, 309: 891–2.

Herrera E, Lasuncion MA, Gomez-Coronado D, Aranda P, Lopez-Luna P, Maier I (1988) Role of lipoprotein lipase activity on lipoprotein metabolism and the fate of circulating triglycerides in pregnancy. American Journal of Obstetrics and Gynecology, 158(6): 1575–83.

Herrera E, Lasuncion MA, Gomez-Coranado L, Martin A, Bonet B (1990) Lipid metabolic interactions in the mother during pregnancy and their fetal repercussions. In Cuezva JM, Pascual-Leon AM, Patel MS (eds) Endocrine and Biochemical Development of the Fetus and Neonate. Plenum Press, New York, pp. 213–30.

Herrera E, Lasuncion MA, Asuncion M (1992) Placental transport of free fatty acids, glycerol, and ketone bodies. In Polin RA, Fox WW (eds) Fetal and Neonatal Physiology. WB Saunders, Philadelphia, pp. 291–8.

Hole RL, Pian-Smith MCM, Sharp GWG (1988) Development of the biphasic response to glucose in fetal and neonatal rat pancreas. American Journal of Physiology, 254: E167–74.

Illingsworth PJ, Jung RT, Howie PW (1986) Diminution in energy expenditure during lactation. British Medical Journal, 292: 437–41.

Issad T, Pastor-Anglada M, Coupe C, Ferre P, Girard J (1990) Glucose metabolism and insulin sensitivity during suckling periods in rats. In Cuezva JM, Pascual-Leon AM, Patel MS (eds) Endocrine and Biochemical Development of the Fetus and Neonate. Plenum Press, New York, pp. 61–6.

Jiang Q, Wakerley JB (1997) The milk-ejection reflex in the peri-partum rat: effects of oestradiol and progesterone on basal milk-ejection frequency and the facilitatory response to central oxytocin. Journal of Neuroendocrinology, 9: 9–16.

Jirikowski GF (1992) Oxytocinergic neuronal systems during mating, pregnancy, parturition and lactation. Annals of the New York Academy of Sciences, 652: 253–70.

Johnston JM, Amico JA (1986) A prospective longitudinal study of the release of oxytocin and prolactin in response to infant suckling in long term lactation. Journal of Clinical Endocrinology and Metabolism, 62(4): 653–7.

Kliegman RM, Sparks JW (1985) Perinatal galactose metabolism. Journal of Pediatrics, 107(6): 831–41.

Ktorza A, Bihoreau M-T, Nurjhan N, Picon L, Girard J (1985) Insulin and glucagon during the perinatal period: secretion and metabolic effects on the liver. Biology of the Neonate, 48: 204–20.

Ladd CO, Owebs MJ, Nemeroff CB (1996) Persistent changes in corticotrophin-releasing factor neuronal systems induced by maternal deprivation. Endocrinology, 137(4): 1212–18.

Lagercrantz H, Marcus C (1992) Sympathoadrenal mechanisms during development. In Polin RA, Fox WW (eds) Fetal and Neonatal Physiology. WB Saunders, Philadelphia, pp. 160–9.

Lagercrantz H, Slotkin TA (1986) The 'stress' of being born. Scientific American, 254: 920–1002.

Lau C, Cameron AM, Antolick LL, Stanton ME (1992) Repeated maternal separation in the neonatal rat: cellular mechanisms contributing to brain growth sparing. Journal of Developmental Physiology, 17: 265–76.

Leung ST, Reynolds TS, Wathes DC (1998) Regulation of oxytocin receptor in the placentome capsule throughout pregnancy in the ewe: the possible role of oestradiol receptor, progesterone receptor and aromatase. Journal of Endocrinology, 158: 173–81.

Lopez-Luna P, Olea J, Herrera E (1994) Effect of starvation on lipoprotein lipase activity in different tissues during gestation in the rat. Biochemica et Biophysica Acta, 1215: 275–9.

Ludington-Hoe SM, Anderson G, Hadeed A (1991) Physiologic responses to skin-to-skin contact in hospitalized premature infants. Journal of Perinatology, 11: 19–24.

Lyonnet S, Coupe C, Girard J, Kahn A, Munnich A (1988) In vivo regulation of glycolytic and gluconeogenic enzyme gene expression in newborn rat liver. Journal of Clinical Investigation, 81: 1682–9.

McCarthy MM, Kow L-M, Pfaffe DW (1992) Speculation concerning the physiological significance of central oxytocin in maternal behaviour. Annals of the New York Academy of Sciences, 652: 70–82.

McKenna JJ, Mosko SS, Richard CA (1997) Bedsharing promotes breastfeeding. Pediatrics, 100(2): 214–19.

Macho L, Fickova M, Zorad S (1995) The effect of early weaning on insulin receptors in rat liver. Endocrine Regulations, 29: 157–62.

Martin AT, Benito CM, Medina JM (1981) Regulation of glycogenolysis in the liver of the newborn rat in vivo, inhibitory effect of glucose. Biochemica et Biophysica Acta, 672: 262–7.

Menon RK, Sperling MA (1988) Carbohydrate metabolism. Seminars in Perinatology, 12(2): 157–62.

Metzinger BE, Ravnikar V, Vilesis RA (1982) 'Accelerated starvation' and the skipped breakfast in late normal pregnancy. Lancet, 1: 588–92.

Mitchell B, Fang X, Wong S (1998) Oxytocin: a paracrine hormone in the regulation of parturition? Reviews of Reproduction, 3: 113–22.

Mueller-Heubach E, Morris M, Rose J (1995) Fetal oxytocin and its extended forms at term with and without labour. American Journal of Obstetrics and Gynecology, 173(2): 375–81.

M'Zali H, Guichard C, Lavau M, Plas C (1997) Time-dependent effects of insulin on lipid synthesis in cultured fetal rat hepatocytes: a comparison between lipogenesis and glycogenesis, Metabolism, 46(4): 345–54.

Nedergaard J, Cannon B (1992) Brown adipose tissue: development and function. In Polin RA, Fox WW (eds) Fetal and Neonatal Physiology. WB Saunders, Philadelphia, pp. 314–25.

Nehlig A, De Vasconcelos AP (1993) Glucose and ketone body utilization by the brain of neonatal rats. Progress in Neurobiology, 40: 163–221.

Neumann I, Douglas AJ, Pittman QJ, Russell JA, Landgraf R (1996) Oxytocin released within the supraoptic nucleus of the rat brain by positive feedback action is involved in parturition-related events. Journal of Neuroendocrinology, 8: 227–33.

Newton N, Newton M (1967) Psychologic aspects of lactation. New England Journal of Medicine, 277(22): 1179–88.

Nissen E, Lija G, Widstrom A-M, Uvnas-Moberg K (1995) Elevation of oxytocin levels early postpartum in women. Acta Obstetrica et Gynaecologica Scandinavica, 74: 530–3.

Nissen E, Lija G, Widstrom A-M, Uvnas-Moberg K (1996) Different patterns of oxytocin, prolactin but not cortisol release during breastfeeding in women delivered by Caesarean section or by the vaginal route. Early Human Development, 45: 103–18.

Odent M (1992) The Nature of Birth and Breastfeeding. Bergin and Garvey, Connecticut.

Odent M (1994) Labouring women are not marathon runners. Midwifery Today, 31: 23–51.

Oliver MH, Harding JE, Breier Evans PC, Gluckman PD (1993) Glucose but not a mixed amino acid infusion regulates plasma insulin-like growth factor-1 concentrations in fetal sheep. Pediatric Research, 34(1): 62–5.

Page EW, Villee CA, Villee DB (1981) Human reproduction: essentials of reproductive and perinatal medicine. WB Saunders, Philadelphia.

Parker SL, Armstrong WE, Sladek CD, Grosvenor CE, Crowley WR (1991) Prolactin stimulates the release of oxytocin in lactating rats: evidence for a physiological role via an action at the neural lobe. Neuroendocrinology, 53: 503–10.

Paterson PJ, Sheath P, Taft P, Wood C (1967) Maternal and foetal ketone concentrations in plasma and urine. Lancet, 1: 862–5.

Petrik J, Arany E, McDonald TJ, Hill DJ (1998) Apoptosis in the pancreatic islet cells of the neonatal rat is associated with a reduced expression of insulin-like growth factor that may act as a survival factor. Endocrinology, 139(6): 2994–3004.

Philipps AF (1992) Carbohydrate metabolism of the fetus. In Polin RA, Fox W (eds) Fetal and Neonatal Physiology. WB Saunders, Philadelphia, pp. 373–84.

Pryor K (1963) Nursing Your Baby. Harper & Row, New York.

Russell JA, Leng G (1998) Sex, parturition and motherhood without oxytocin? Journal of Endocrinology, 157: 343–59.

Sabata V, Wolf H, Lausmann S (1968) The role of free fatty acids, glycerol, ketone bodies and glucose in the energy metabolism of mother and fetus during delivery. Biology of the Neonate, 13: 7–17.

Sadava D, Frykman P, Harris Emajerus D, Mustard J, Bernard B (1992) Development of enzymes of glycolysis and gluconeogenesis in human fetal liver. Biology of the Neonate, 62: 89–95.

Samson WK, Lumpkin MD, McCann SM (1986) Evidence for a physiological role for oxytocin in the control of prolactin secretion. Endocrinology, 119(2): 554–60.

Sarvetnick N (ed.) (1997) Pancreatic Growth and Regeneration. Karger, Basel.

Scaglia L, Cahill CJ, Finegood DT, Bonner-Weir S (1997) Apoptosis participates in the remodeling of the endocrine pancreas in the neonatal rat. Endocrinology, 138(4): 1736–41.

Schambaugh GE (1985) Ketone body metabolism in the mother and fetus. FASEB Journal, 44: 2347–51.

Seccombe DW, Harding PGR, Possmayer F (1977) Fetal utilization of maternally derived ketone bodies for lipogenesis in the rat. Biochemica et Biophysica Acta, 488: 402–16.

Simmons M, Jones MD, Battaglia FC, Meschia G (1978) Insulin effects on fetal glucose utilization. Pediatric Research, 12: 90–2.

Smith MA, Kim S-Y, van Oers HJJ, Levine S (1997) Maternal deprivation and stress induced immediate early genes in the infant rat brain. Endocrinology, 138(11): 4622–8.

Sorenson RL, Clarke Brelje T, Roth C (1993) Effects of steroid and lactogenic hormones on islets of Langerhans: a new hypothesis for the role of pregnancy steroids in the adaptation of islets to pregnancy. Endocrinology, 133(5): 2227–34.

Sparks JW (1992) Galactose and fructose. In Polin RA, Fox WW (eds), Fetal and Neonatal Physiology. WB Saunders, Philadelphia, pp. 384–90.

Sperling MA (1994) Carbohydrate metabolism: insulin and glucagon. In Tulchinsky D, Little AB (eds) Maternal and Fetal Endocrinology. WB Saunders, Philadelphia, pp. 379–400.

Sperling MA, DeLamater PV, Phelps D et al (1974) Spontaneous and amino acid stimulated glucagon secretion in the immediate postnatal period: relation to glucose and insulin. Journal of Clinical Investigation, 53: 1159–66.

Steingrimsdottir T, Ronquist G, Ulmsten U (1993) Energy economy in the pregnant human uterus at term: studies on arteriovenous differences in metabolites of carbohydrate, fat and nucleotides. European Journal of Obstetrics, Gynaecology and Reproductive Biology, 51: 209–15.

Stephenson T, Stammers J, Hull D (1993) Placental transfer of free fatty acids: importance of fetal albumen concentration and acid–base status. Biology of the Neonate, 63: 273–80.

Symonds ME, Bird JA, Clarke L, Gate JJ, Lomax MA (1995) Nutrition, temperature and homeostasis during perinatal development. Experimental Physiology, 80: 907–40.

Thomas A, Crowley RS, Amico JA (1995) Effect of progesterone on hypothalamic oxytocin messenger ribonucleic acid levels in the lactating rat. Endocrinology, 136(10): 4188–94.

Uvnas-Moberg K (1989) The gastrointestinal tract in growth and reproduction. Scientific American (Jul): 60–5.

Uvnas-Moberg K (1996) Neuroendocrinology of the mother–child interaction. Trends in Endocrinology and Metabolism, 7(4): 126–31.

Uvnas-Moberg K, Winberg J (1989) Role of sensory stimulation in energy economy of mother and infant with particular regard to the gastrointestinal endocrine system. In Lebenthal E (ed.) Textbook of Gastroenterology and Nutrition in Infancy. Raven Press, New York, pp. 53–61.

Uvnas-Moberg K, Bruzelius G, Alster P, Lundberg T (1993) The antinociceptive effect of non-noxious sensory stimulation is mediated partly through oxytocinergic mechanisms. Acta Physiologica Scandinavica, 149: 199–204.

Uvnas-Moberg K, Alster P, Petersson M, Sohlstrom A, Bjorkstrand E (1998) Postnatal oxytocin injections cause sustained weight gain and increased nociceptive thresholds in male and female rats. Pediatric Research, 43(3): 344–8.

van Ores HJJ, de Kloet ER, Li C, Levine S (1998) The ontogeny of glucocorticoid feedback: influence of maternal deprivation. Endocrinology, 139(6): 2838–46.

Varendi H, Porter RH, Winberg J (1994) Does the newborn baby find the nipple by smell? Lancet, 344: 989–90.

Wakerley JB, Clarke G, Summerlee G (1994) Milk ejection and its control. In Knobil E, Neill JD, Greenwald GS *et al* (eds) The Physiology of Reproduction. Raven Press, New York, pp. 1131–377.

Wedenberg K, Ronquist G, Waldenstrom A, Ulmsten U (1990) Low energy charge in human uterine muscle. Biochemica et Biophysica Acta, 1033: 31–4.

Widmaier EP (1990) Changes in responsiveness of the hypothalamic-pituitary-adrenocortical axis to 2-deoxy-D-glucose in developing rats. Endocrinology, 126(6): 3116–23.

Widmaier EP (1991) Endocrine control of glucose homeostasis in mammals: food for thought. Molecular and Cellular Endocrinology, 75: C1–6.

Williams DH (1992) Ketone body production and metabolism in the fetus and newborn. In Polin RA, Fox WW (eds) Fetal and Neonatal Physiology. WB Saunders, Philadelphia, pp. 330–4.

Yuan ZF, Pan J-T (1996) Stimulatory effect of central oxytocin on tuberoinfundibular dopaminergic neuron activity and inhibition on prolactin secretion: neurochemical and electrophysiological studies. Endocrinology, 137(10): 4120–5.

Zhu Y, Goff JP, Reinhardt TA, Horst RL (1998) Pregnancy and lactation increases vitamin D-dependent intestinal membrane calcium adenosine triphosphatase and calcium binding protein messenger ribonucleic acid expression. Endocrinology, 139(8): 3520–4.

Chapter 5

Breastfeeding update

Sally Inch

■ Introduction

Although there have been numerous studies since the publication of 'Post-natal care relating to breastfeeding' (Inch 1990) that have added to our understanding of the physiology of lactation, the fundamental principles of breastfeeding – good attachment and unrestricted feeding frequency and duration – have not changed. This chapter will therefore concentrate on how these two fundamentals can be enhanced in a hospital setting.

It considers the quality and design of research studies that have demonstrated the superiority of breastfeeding over bottle-feeding.

On the strength of the evidence of its superiority, the chapter goes on to examine the practical application of the WHO/UNICEF Baby Friendly Hospital Initiative and the implementation of the Ten Steps to Successful Breastfeeding (WHO 1989).

■ It is assumed that you are already aware of the following:

● The anatomy of the breast;

● The physiology of lactation;

and that you have read the previous chapter on breastfeeding in the Midwifery Practice series (Inch 1990).

■ Health benefits

☐ Breastfeeding and babies

Few would argue with the concept that, in countries where bottle-feeding cannot be safely carried out (because of a lack of fuel, a lack of clean water, an inability to afford an appropriate milk powder in sufficient quantity, an inability to read the instructions for reconstitution and so on), breastfeeding is a much better option. UNICEF estimates that one and a half million babies die every year from unsafe bottle-feeding, most of the deaths arising from diarrhoeal disease.

However, the assumption that 'breast is best' for babies born in industrialised countries was challenged in 1986 by Bauchner *et al*. They examined the extent to which 20 studies that claimed to have demonstrated an association between breastfeeding and a reduced incidence of infection met what they considered to be the four important methodological standards that related to both their scientific validity and generalisability. These were as follows:

- *The avoidance of detection bias in the study design*
  It is rarely either ethical or possible to conduct randomised controlled trials of infant feeding methods, so most studies are either observational cohort studies (either retrospective or prospective) or case-control studies.

  Bauchner *et al* (1986) considered that the only way in which the outcome event (infection) could be detected with equal readiness in both groups was if 'active surveillance' had taken place. This means making contact with all the mothers and babies in both groups at frequent, prescribed intervals. Retrospective studies were therefore automatically excluded.

- *Adequate control for confounding variables*
  In order to be able to attribute differences in the rate of infection to the method of feeding, either other factors that might also affect the incidence must have been present equally in both groups (by matching), or adjustment must have been made in the statistical analyses for those important differences that were present. The most important confounding variable was considered to be socioeconomic status, but size of family, maternal smoking and maternal education were also regarded as significant variables.

- *Clearly defined outcome events*
  In order to be generalisable, the study needed to define precisely what, for example, constituted 'diarrhoea' or an 'upper respiratory tract infection'.

- *A clear definition of what is mean by 'breastfeeding'*
  The usual categories are (a) exclusively breastfed, (b) partially breastfed, and (c) not breastfed. The length of time for which a baby remained in categories (a) and (b) might also be important. Bauchner *et al* did not specify exactly what these definitions should be, and there is unfortunately considerable scope for interpretation, particularly in the 'partially breastfed' category. This makes comparison between studies problematic.

Of the 20 studies examined using these criteria, only 2 out of the 14 cohort studies met all four standards; a further 3 met three out of the four standards. None of the 6 case-control studies met all four standards, and only 1 met three of the four. Of the six studies that met three or four of the standards, only two found that breastfeeding exerted a protective effect.

As well as suggesting that all subsequent studies be designed with their standards in mind, Bauchner *et al* (1986) made further suggestions. They considered that variations in the duration of breastfeeding, the amount of breast milk received and the length of time for which breastfeeding was exclusive might influence the extent to which breastfeeding exerted a protective effect. They wondered if there was a threshold level of either the amount or the duration at which breastfeeding became protective.

Bauchner *et al* (1986) made a further point in relation to the importance of 'power calculations'. The ability (or power) of a study to detect a real difference (if one exists) will depend on the prevalence of the outcome event in the control group and the number of subjects recruited to each group. The actual number needed in the sample will depend on the size of difference in the outcome event between the control and intervention group that the researchers consider clinically relevant and therefore wish to be able to detect.

Two years later, in a review of the association between breastfeeding and atopic disease, Kramer (1988) described a set of 12 methodological standards. To those listed by Bauchner *et al* he added:

- A non-reliance on maternal recall;

- A blind ascertainment of infant feeding history (that is, details being taken without knowing whether the infant was affected by atopic disease);

- A blind ascertainment of outcome (that is, a determination of the existence or severity of atopic disease without knowing how the infant had been fed);

- Information on the severity of outcome;

- The age at onset of the outcome;

- An assessment of the dose–response effect;

- An assessment of the effect on children at high risk of developing atopic disease (that is, where there is a strong family history of this);

- Adequate statistical power.

One of the first studies to be published that addressed all of Bauchner's criteria was that of Howie *et al* (1990), which was designed to assess the relationship between breastfeeding and infant illness in the first 2 years of life, with particular reference to gastrointestinal illness.

Sample size was determined using the difference in the rate of gastrointestinal illness between breastfed and bottle-fed infants detected by Fergusson *et al* (1981) of 8.7 per cent. To be 90 per cent certain of detecting a difference of this magnitude at the 5 per cent level of significance ($p < 0.05$), 280 infants would be needed in each group. Seven hundred and fifty were thus recruited, 618 still remaining at 2 years, a reflection of the stability of the study population (Dundee).

Detection bias was minimised by a combination of 'hot pursuit' and 'cold pursuit'. All the mothers and babies in the study were interviewed by health visitors at prescribed intervals (2 weeks and 1, 2, 3, 4, 6, 9, 12, 15, 18, 21 and 24 months), and the medical records were searched retrospectively. Thus, the only episodes of illness that would have been undetected would be those that the mother had forgotten and the GP had failed to record.

Confounding variables were established by applying discriminant (regressional) analysis to over 40 variables. Ultimately, only social class, maternal smoking and maternal age remained.

Outcome events were defined using Chandra's criteria (1979). Gastrointestinal disease was thus defined as vomiting and/or diarrhoea lasting 48 hours or more.

Breastfeeding was defined and the method of feeding was determined by asking the mother (at each visit), 'how did you feed your baby yesterday?' and was thus not based on historical recall.

For the purposes of comparison, mothers were divided into four groups: *full breastfeeders,* who breastfed for 13 weeks or more and gave no supplements before 13 weeks; *partial breastfeeders,* who breastfed for at least 13 weeks but also gave supplements before 13 weeks; *early weaners,* who began breastfeeding but ceased completely before 13 weeks, and those who *bottle fed from birth.*

The observed incidence of gastrointestinal disease at 3 months in babies whose mothers were defined as full breastfeeders was 2.2 per cent. In babies who were bottle-fed at birth, it was 20 per cent. After adjusting for confounding variables, the rates were 3.5 per cent and 16 per cent respectively. Furthermore, a significant difference in the incidence persisted well beyond the first year (Figure 5.1).

Seven years later, Wilson *et al* (1998) were able to follow up 545 of the babies (now children) from the original study and obtain data on respiratory illness, growth and body composition and blood pressure. Significant differences could still be demonstrated between the children, depending on whether they had been exclusively breastfed for at least 15 weeks or bottle-fed, breastfed children having significantly lower blood pressure and a lower incidence of respiratory illnesses. Early solid feeding was associated with an increased incidence of wheeze, increased weight and a higher percentage of body fat.

Studies published since 1986 that have met at least three of the four criteria described by Bauchner *et al* (1986) have subsequently provided strong evidence that breastfeeding protects infants from diarrhoeal disease,

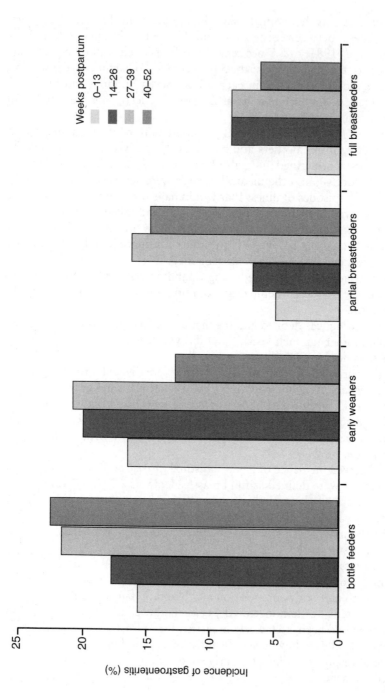
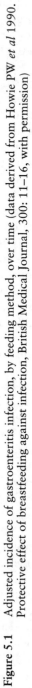

Figure 5.1 Adjusted incidence of gastroenteritis infection, by feeding method, over time (data derived from Howie PW *et al* 1990. Protective effect of breastfeeding against infection, British Medical Journal, 300: 11–16, with permission)

lower respiratory tract disease and otitis media. Well-conducted studies have also demonstrated a protective effect against urinary tract infection, diabetes mellitus, necrotising enterocolitis and sudden infant death. Children born into families with a history of atopic disease are at reduced risk of eczema and respiratory wheeze if they are breastfed. Both term and preterm infants have higher cognitive development scores if they are breastfed rather than bottle-fed.

These studies have been critically reviewed by Heinig and Dewey (1996) Woolridge (1996) and the NHS Centre for Reviews and Dissemination (MIDIRS/NHS Centre for Reviews and Dissemination 1997).

☐ Breast milk and babies

One of the very few areas in which it has been possible to conduct a randomised controlled trial of breast milk versus breast milk substitutes has been that of special or intensive care nurseries, where mothers have been unable to supply sufficient, if any, of their own breast milk for their babies, and whose babies could therefore be randomised to receive either donated breast milk or formula milk, either exclusively or to make up the shortfall.

In the two multicentre trials conducted by Lucas and Cole (1990), 926 infants were assigned to their early diet, receiving donor breast milk, term formula or preterm formula as a supplement to maternal breast milk in one trial, while in the second trial, involving babies whose mothers had elected not to provide any of their own milk, babies received either donor milk or preterm formula. Necrotising enterocolitis developed in 51 (5.5 per cent). Mortality was 26 per cent in stringently confirmed cases. The 253 infants fed only human milk ranged from those fed exclusively pasteurised donor breast milk to those fed almost entirely on raw maternal milk, but the incidence of necrotising enterocolitis in this subgroup was not affected by the type of breast milk consumed. The rate of necrotising enterocolitis did not differ between the two types of formula milk in the subgroup (236 infants) who received either term or preterm formula as their sole diet. Thus, the whole population could be divided into three large diet groups for comparison: formula only (236), formula plus breast milk (437) and breast milk only (253).

Confirmed cases of necrotising enterocolitis occurred in 7.2 per cent of the formula-only group, 2.5 per cent of the formula plus mother's milk and 1.2 per cent of the breast milk-only group. After adjustment for a wide range of factors known to be associated with the disease, confirmed necrotising enterocolitis was 10 times as common in babies fed formula only as in those fed breast milk only (and 3.5 times higher than in those fed both formula and breast milk). The difference was even more dramatic when the length of gestation was considered: beyond 30 weeks' gestation, the incidence of necrotising enterocolitis in formula-fed infants was 20 times as great as in those fed some breast milk.

☐ *Milk banking*

The study by Lucas and Cole (1990) powerfully confirmed data from other studies suggesting that there was an increased risk of necrotising enterocolitis if infants were exclusively formula fed. Unfortunately, this study was published too late to prevent the mass closure of human milk banks in the UK in the late 1980s, driven by the fear of HIV transmission (despite the work of Eglin and Wilkinson, 1987, that had demonstrated the effectiveness of pasteurisation in destroying the virus if present) and the rising popularity of preterm formulas. By the early 1990s, there were only six milk banks left in the UK (Weaver 1996). This number has now slowly risen, encouraged by the publication of the British Paediatric Association guidelines for human milk banks in 1994, currently (1999) standing at 13; all but two of these (Glasgow and Huddersfield) are in the Midlands or south of England.

In 1998's Breastfeeding Week, the UK Human Milk Banking Association was launched, spearheaded by the Queen Charlotte's and Chelsea Hospital Milk Bank. The hope is to make human milk more readily available to preterm infants and to encourage and support the setting up of new milk banks.

☐ **Breastfeeding and mothers**

The methodological criteria set out by Bauchner *et al* (1986) are equally important with respect to studies that have examined the effects of breastfeeding in relation to the mother. However, far more of these studies are retrospective in relation to the information provided on the duration and/or exclusivity of breastfeeding that took place, sometimes several decades before the outcome in question.

Critical reviews of studies that met at least three of Bauchner's four criteria have been published by Heinig and Dewey (1997) and the NHS Centre for Reviews and Dissemination (1997). These conclude that there is considerable evidence to suggest significant health advantages for mothers who breastfeed their infants, most notably a reduction in the incidence of premenopausal breast, ovarian and endometrial cancers.

This large and growing body of research evidence that breastfeeding is significantly and demonstrably better able to nourish the newborn and protect the health of both the mother and her baby than any breast milk substitute has refuelled efforts to protect, promote and support breastfeeding world wide.

■ The 'birth' of the Baby Friendly Hospital Initiative

In 1989 the World Health Organisation and UNICEF published a 32-page joint statement entitled *Protecting, Promoting and Supporting Breast-feeding – the Special Role of the Maternity Services*. This document contained the Ten Steps to Successful Breastfeeding and formed the back-bone of the global enterprise the Baby Friendly Hospital Initiative, which was launched in Ankara in 1991 and is directed towards increasing both the number of babies that are breastfed from birth and the length of time for which they are breastfed.

The research basis for the Ten Steps – 'Evidence for the ten steps to successful breastfeeding' – has been recently published (Vallenas & Savage 1998). The references to support the section below on the 'The Ten Steps in Practice' are all to be found in that publication and will not be repeated here.

Throughout the world, the Baby Friendly Hospital Initiative addresses one of the main obstacles to successful breastfeeding – health care practices that interfere with the establishment of breastfeeding. Fully implementing the Ten Steps (Figure 5.2) and the International Code on the Marketing of Breastmilk Substitutes removes these obstacles.

There are now tens of thousands of hospitals world wide that have implemented both the Ten Steps and the International Code on the Marketing of Breastmilk Substitutes, and thus achieved Baby Friendly status. With this has come a rise in both the initiation rate and duration of breastfeeding.

UNICEF (1998) reports that, in Chile in 1985, only 4 per cent of babies were breastfed; by 1996, this figure had risen to 40 per cent. In Cuba, 63 per cent of babies were breastfed before the introduction of the Baby Friendly Hospital Initiative; 6 years later, this had risen to 98 per cent, the duration of breastfeeding also having increased. By the end of 1996, China had over 6300 hospitals designated as baby friendly, with 48–68 per cent of babies reported as being exclusively breastfed for 4 months.

☐ The UK Baby Friendly Initiative

In 1994 the Initiative was extended to the UK, where the UNICEF UK Baby Friendly Initiative exists to support health professionals who wish to imple-ment best practice standards in all health care settings and to ensure that all mothers are able to make informed decisions concerning feeding and caring for their babies.

For hospitals, best practice is encapsulated by the Ten Steps, and for community settings by the Seven Point Plan (launched during Breastfeeding Week in May 1998), which mirrors the Ten Steps and extends the principles into community health care settings.

TEN STEPS TO SUCCESSFUL BREASTFEEDING

Every facility providing maternity services and care for newborn infants should:

1. Have a written breastfeeding policy that is routinely communicated to all health care staff.

2. Train all health care staff in skills necessary to implement the breastfeeding policy.

3. Inform all pregnant women about the benefits and management of breastfeeding.

4. Help the mother to initiate breastfeeding within half an hour of birth.

5. Show mothers how to breastfeed and how to maintain lactation even if they are separated from their infants.

6. Give newborn infants no food or drink other than breast milk, unless medically indicated.

7. Practice rooming-in: allowing mothers and infants to remain together 24 hours a day.

8. Encourage breastfeeding on demand.

9. Give no artificial teats or pacifiers (also called dummies or soothers) to breastfeeding infants.

10. Foster the establishment of breastfeeding support groups and refer mothers to them on discharge from hospital or clinic.

Figure 5.2   Ten Steps to Successful Breastfeeding

■ The Ten Steps in Practice

The framework for implementing the Ten Steps is contained in step 1 – providing a written policy and a mechanism for communicating this policy to both the staff and the women using the health care facility. The presentation may vary, but it must be a policy rather than guidelines so that it is clear that all staff must follow it. Once it is in place, some form of auditing is necessary to ensure that the policy is being put into practice.

The policy should address all Ten Steps and also include explicit guidance to staff on the implementation of the International Code on the Marketing of Breastmilk Substitutes. This means no advertising of breast milk substitutes, however unintentional, in any part of the facility, on any document or in the hands of any member of staff.

Hospitals should be able to demonstrate that they receive no free or discounted breast milk substitutes (in line with UK law), and community-based health care facilities are precluded from selling such substitutes at a reduced rate on their premises.

A great many of the health professionals currently practising received very little information on breastfeeding management as part of their basic training, yet they are expected to provide skilled help and appropriate advice to mothers. Step 2 acknowledges that basic training may have been inadequate and requires that in-service training not only is mandatory, but will also improve practical skills as well as knowledge. The decision to breast- or bottle-feed will profoundly affect the future health of the mother and her baby, and should be based on something stronger than the odd magazine feature, anecdotes or the experience of friends.

Step 3 requires that all pregnant women are able to make a fully informed choice. They need to know that, compared with a fully breastfed baby, a baby who is bottle-fed from birth is:

- Five times more likely to be hospitalised with gastroenteritis (within the first 3 months of life);

- Five times more likely to suffer from a urinary infection (within the first 6 months of life);

- Twice as likely to suffer from chest infections (within the first 7 years of life);

- Twice as likely to suffer from ear infection (within the first year of life);

- Twice as likely to develop atopic disease where there is a family history of this;

- Up to 20 times more likely to develop necrotising enterocolitis if born prematurely.

The purpose of this information is not to frighten women into breastfeeding but to make sure that they are aware that infant feeding is not just a matter of choosing between two equivalent methods that can safely be determined purely on the basis of what is socially and culturally expedient.

Although there are a variety of leaflets detailing the health benefits of breastfeeding, the best way to communicate information to pregnant women is probably to provide them with an opportunity to talk about it, preferably on a one-to-one basis, some time during the second half of pregnancy, in the same way that birth plans are often discussed.

It is also vital that pregnant women are made aware that breastfeeding is not instinctive but a skill that has to be learned. At some point during the antenatal period, women should be made aware of how a baby feeds and why good attachment and baby-led feeding are so important in establishing and maintaining good milk supply and preventing problems such as engorgement and sore nipples. Any written information given to the woman as a reminder of the points raised in discussion should be brief, accurate and easy to read.

Well-designed antenatal education classes have been shown to be particularly effective in building a woman's confidence and skills, and if the information can be shared with her partner, relatives or female peers, it may help them to help her in the early days and weeks of the baby's life.

The practical aspects of making up bottle feeds are best taught individually and according to need, after the baby is born, and should not form part of an antenatal class.

Step 4 requires that, unless the circumstances of the delivery dictate otherwise, all mothers, regardless of feeding intention, should have the opportunity of immediate skin-to-skin contact with their babies and that this contact should continue for as long as the mother wants. Babies who are kept in their mother's arms after delivery are observed to cry less than those placed in a cot, and many mothers report that prolonged contact and early breastfeeding helped them to feel emotionally close to their baby. The warmth of the mother's body will maintain her baby's temperature, particularly if the mother is covered, and breastfeeding can be initiated as soon as the mother and baby are ready. Help should be given if the mother wishes it, and further help should be offered with breastfeeding within 6 hours of delivery.

Good attachment of the baby at the breast is the essence of successful and satisfying breastfeeding. However, most women do not automatically know how to attach their babies well, and it should not be assumed, even with mothers who have fed before, that no help will be needed at the beginning. Teaching a mother the principles of good attachment and guiding her as she learns to put them into practice are the most valuable things that a health professional can do for a new mother. Almost all postnatal breastfeeding problems can be prevented if the baby is able to feed effectively and efficiently from the beginning. Good attachment is evident from the rhythm of the feed, the baby's relaxed body and the fact that he causes his mother no discomfort and terminates the feed spontaneously.

Hand-expressing is a useful technique for all breastfeeding mothers to learn. It helps them to understand how their breasts function and gives them the confidence that their body is working normally. In the early days, a very full breast can be softened gently to enable the baby to attach more easily, and later on a mother can express milk for someone else to give to her baby if they are separated for any reason.

If the mother and baby are separated shortly after birth, because the baby is preterm or ill for example, help and support with expressing colostrum, and later milk, is essential. The earlier the mother can begin to express and the more often she can do it, the greater the likelihood of establishing breastfeeding. Although most mothers find that colostrum is more easily expressed by hand, automatic electric pumps may be faster and easier once there is a greater volume of milk, particularly if pumping will have to be continued for some time. Many mothers in this situation find that expressing both breasts at the same time, or double pumping, helps them to produce more milk in less time. Mothers who are expressing to establish or maintain their lactation should be advised to do so at least 6–8 times in 24 hours, including once at night, although the intervals between sessions do not need to be regular.

Step 6 requires that a healthy term breastfed baby is given no food or drink other than breast milk. He is born with adequate reserves of food and fluid in his body, and the hormones present at birth reduce fluid loss in the first 2 days of life. The colostrum the baby obtains from his mother's breast provides him with all that he needs until her milk 'comes in'. Thereafter, a baby who is meeting his calorie requirements from breast milk and growing well is certainly meeting his fluid requirements. Giving a newborn baby supplements, even of water, increases the risk of infection, reduces the frequency of breastfeeding and hence the amount of nipple stimulation and, later, milk removal. Unless supplements are medically indicated, they may also make the mother feel that she is somehow inadequate.

Guidelines on hypoglycaemia should reflect the fact that healthy term newborns are well able to maintain an adequate blood sugar level even if they feed infrequently, and the measurement of blood glucose level is unnecessary in such infants. A recent research-based WHO publication (Williams 1996) provided the foundation for the consensus group that produced national guidelines in 1997 (NCT 1997), and these should form the basis of all local policies.

If there is concern about the infrequency of the feeds in the first 24 hours, particularly if the baby's mother has received narcotics in labour, the baby can be gently roused, perhaps by changing his nappy, and offered the breast. If it is not possible to wake the baby sufficiently to attach to the breast, hand-expressed colostrum can be given to the baby by syringe or cup so that none is wasted.

Rooming-in is important for all mothers, no matter how the baby is fed, and no baby should be routinely removed from the mother's bedside at night. Routine nursery care reduces the interaction between mother and infant and may make the mother feel less confident in responding appropriately to her baby when she goes home. Controlled studies have shown that mothers and babies who remain together throughout the night sleep as well, if not better, than those who are separated, and the mother is better able to respond to the baby's cues for feeding if she is close by (Vallenas & Savage 1998). If an otherwise well baby develops jaundice that requires phototherapy treatment, this should be carried out by the mother's bedside, or as close by as possible, so that breastfeeding is not interrupted.

Breastfeeding mothers should be encouraged to breastfeed their babies whenever they want and to allow their correctly attached baby to feed until he terminates the feed spontaneously. The restrictions on the duration and the interval between feeds that were introduced at the beginning of the 20th century, in the mistaken belief that they would prevent gastrointestinal disturbances in the baby and sore nipples in the mother, have subsequently been shown to interfere with the establishment of breastfeeding, causing engorgement, poor milk production and poor weight gain in the infant.

Dummies are usually used to calm an infant without giving a feed. The mother of a newborn baby that can only be settled with the use of a dummy probably needs further help with attaching her baby to her breast correctly. If a dummy is used as a substitute for improving breastfeeding technique, breast stimulation and milk removal will be reduced. In the medium term, this may adversely affect the mother's milk supply and thus her baby's nutritional needs, and in the longer term it may allow ovulation and menstruation to return earlier than it might otherwise have done. The use of dummies has been shown to be associated with a reduced duration of breastfeeding.

If a breastfed baby needs to be given expressed colostrum, it is more practical to give this small amount by syringe or dropper so that none is wasted. Preterm infants are often able to cup feed before they are able to breastfeed, and cup feeding might therefore reduce the need for nasogastric feeds. Preterm infants show more signs of stress (such as increased oxygen use) when fed by bottle compared with breastfeeding, and cup feeding might be preferable to bottle-feeding when the mother is absent from the unit. There is some evidence that the use of cups rather than bottles for preterm infants is associated with an increased incidence of breastfeeding on discharge home (Lang *et al* 1994). However, the frequently used term 'nipple confusion', which suggests that an otherwise normal term newborn baby is unable to adapt his suckling technique to feed from a bottle, or that having done so he will be unable to feed well from the breast, has no basis in fact (Fisher & Inch 1996).

Nipple shields are of very limited value in solving breastfeeding problems. They should never be used before the mother has an established milk supply as it is unlikely that the baby will be able to draw enough colostrum through the shield to meet his needs. If the problem that they are being used to circumvent is difficult attachment as a result of inelastic breast tissue, the mother would be better advised to express by hand or with an electric pump as this is more likely to result in softening and stretching the breast tissue than is the use of a shield. Although there are exceptions, it is unlikely that the baby will be able to use the breast effectively through a shield, and this may result in engorgement or mastitis in the mother and poor weight gain in the baby.

Implementing step 10 ensures that mothers leave hospital knowing that help and support are available in the community. Up-to-date contact details should be given to the mother separately and in writing. She should be made aware of the more informal local groups that exist to support mothers and babies generally, and breastfeeding mothers in particular, and should be given contact numbers for the four national lay groups that provide breast-feeding support and advice: the National Childbirth Trust, the Association of Breastfeeding Mothers, the National Breastfeeding Network and the La Leche League.

When the community midwife passes the care of the mother and baby to the health visitor, giving brief details relating to the mother's breastfeeding experience will help to avoid conflicting information and allow a more seamless delivery of care. The ongoing problem of conflicting advice was highlighted yet again in the recently published Audit Commission (1998) report *First Class Delivery*. Evidence from over 2400 women revealed that, in relation to breastfeeding, 'the midwife at the hospital said one thing, the midwife who came to see them at home another and the health visitor said something different again' (Nolan 1998, p. 4). Yet continued (consistent) support by both health professionals and peer group counsellors has been repeatedly shown to increase the time for which breastfeeding is continued (Inch & Renfrew 1989; Vallenas & Savage 1998). The gulf between these two findings can only be bridged by improving the quality of both the practical and the theoretical training that health professionals receive.

This would surely be aided by measures taken (at government level) to improve the chronic understaffing of many UK maternity units. The findings of the expert committee convened in 1997 by the Secretary of State for Health and chaired by Sir Donald Acheson were revealed at the annual Edwin Chadwick lecture in November 1998 (Laurance 1998). The committee's remit had been to examine what could be done to close the health gap between rich and poor, which had widened during the preceding 17 years of Tory rule. Using a complex formula to assess the strength of the evidence, the scale of probable benefit, the fit with government policy and the ease and cost of implementation, they produced a list of 10 interventions most likely to help the poor more than the rich (thus closing the gap) and unlikely to do harm. The sixth on the list was 'Support around childbirth to promote breastfeeding... for which there is... good evidence of long term benefits'. It will be interesting to see how this recommendation is put into practice.

■ Recommendations for clinical practice in the light of currently available evidence

1. There is overwhelming evidence that it is in the best interests of both the mother and her newborn baby that she should breastfeed. No health professional should give the impression to a pregnant or newly delivered woman that it does not really matter whether she breastfeeds or bottle-feeds her child. It is patronising (and dishonest) to withhold the facts to protect the woman from 'feeling guilty'. Curiously enough, health

professionals do not seem to have the same scruples when it comes to giving information about smoking in pregnancy.

2. Women elect to bottle feed their babies for a variety of reasons: their medical condition may preclude breastfeeding, their social circumstances may make breastfeeding and working very difficult, or they may feel that they will not get the help or support from their partner, peers or relatives that they will need to breastfeed happily.

3. Having ascertained that the mother has made an informed choice, health professionals have a duty to support the mother in her choice and assist her to bottle-feed safely. This should include ensuring that she knows how to prepare feeds accurately and sterilise equipment effectively, as well as observing her bottle-feeding technique.

4. It is in the best interests of all mothers and babies that maternity hospitals fully implement the Ten Steps to Successful Breastfeeding. This can be done independently of applying for Baby Friendly status.

■ Practice check

- Does your hospital have a written breastfeeding policy? Is it in line with the Ten Steps to Successful Breastfeeding?

- Is practice in relation to breastfeeding audited regularly in your hospital?

- Does your hospital provide adequate in-service training in the practical as well as the theoretical aspects of breastfeeding?

- Do you ensure that all breastfeeding women know how to hand-express?

- Does your hospital have a milk bank? (If not, could you set one up?)

- Does your hospital have a designated breastfeeding advisor/infant feeding specialist (DoH 1995)?

- How do you minimise the risk of giving conflicting advice to breast-feeding women?

■ References

Audit Commission (1998) First class delivery: A National Survey of Women's Views of Maternity Care. Audit Commission, London.
Bauchner H, Leventhal JM, Shapiro ED (1986) Studies of breast-feeding and infection – how good is the evidence? Journal of the American Medical Association, 256(7): 887–92.

British Paediatric Association (1994) Guidelines for the Establishment and Operation of Human Milk Banks in the UK. Standing Committee of Nutrition of the British Paediatric Association, London.

Chandra RK (1979) Prospective studies of the effect of breast feeding on incidence of infection and allergy. Acta Paediatrica Scandanavica, 68: 691–94.

Department of Health (1995) Breastfeeding: Good Practice Guidance to the NHS. Prepared in consultation with the National Breastfeeding Working Group. HMSO, London.

Eglin RP, Wilkinson AR (1987) HIV infection and pasteurisation of breastmilk. Lancet, 8541: 1092–3.

Fergusson DM, Horwood JL, Shannon FT, Taylor B (1981) Breastfeeding, gastrointestinal disease and lower respiratory illness in the first two years. Australian Paediatric Journal, 17: 191–5.

Fisher C, Inch S (1996) Nipple confusion – who is confused? Journal of Paediatrics, 129(1): 174.

Heinig MJ, Dewey KG (1996) Health advantages of breast feeding for infants: a critical review. Nutrition Research Review, 9: 89–110.

Heinig MJ, Dewey KG (1997) Health effects of breast feeding for mothers: a critical review. Nutrition Research Review, 10: 35–56.

Howie PW, Forsyth JS, Ogston SA, Clark A, Florey CV (1990) Protective effect of breast feeding against infection. British Medical Journal, 300: 11–16.

Inch S (1990) Postnatal care relating to breastfeeding. In Alexander J, Levy V, Roch S (eds) Postnatal care – a Research Based Approach. Macmillan, Basingstoke, pp. 18–44.

Inch S, Renfrew MJ (1989) Common breastfeeding problems. In Chalmers I, Enkin M, Keirse MJNC (eds) Effective Care in Pregnancy and Childbirth. Oxford University Press, Oxford, pp. 375–87.

Kramer MS (1988) Does breast feeding help protect against atopic disease? Biology, methodology and a golden jubilee of controversy. Journal of Pediatrics, 112: 181–90.

Lang S, Lawrence CJ, Orme RL'E (1994) Cup feeding: an alternative method of infant feeding. Archives of Disease in Childhood, 71: 365–9.

Laurance J (1998) Experts' 10 steps to health equality. Independent, 12 November, p. 14.

Lucas A, Cole TJ (1990) Breast milk and neonatal necrotising entercolitis. Lancet, 336: 519–23.

National Childbirth Trust (1997) Hypoglycaemia of the Newborn: Guidelines for Appropriate Blood Glucose Screening and Treatment of Breastfed and Bottle Fed Babies in the United Kingdom. National Childbirth Trust, Glasgow.

MIDIRS/NHS Centre for Reviews and Dissemination (1997) Informed choice paired leaflets for health professionals and for pregnant women. Leaflet 5: i) Breastfeeding or bottle feeding: helping women to chose, ii) Feeding your baby – breast or bottle? MIDIRS, Bristol.

Nolan M (1998) Listening to women. Practising Midwife 1(3): 4 Editorial.

UNICEF (1998) The State of the World's Children 1998. Oxford University Press, Oxford.

Vallenas C, Savage F (1998) Evidence for the ten steps to successful breastfeeding. Division of Child Health and Development, WHO, Geneva.

Weaver G (1996) The history of milk banking. Address given at the Symposium on Milk Banking – Past, Present and Future. Queen Charlotte's and Chelsea Hospital, 30 September.

Williams A (1996) Hypoglycaemia and the Newborn. WHO, Geneva.

Wilson AC, Forsyth JS, Greene SA, Irvine L, Hau C, Howie PW (1998) Relationship of infant diet to childhood health: seven year follow up of cohort of children in Dundee Infant Feeding Study. British Medical Journal, 316: 21–5.

Woolridge M (1996) Information sheet on the health benefits of breastfeeding. Compiled for and obtainable from: UNICEF UK Baby Friendly Initiative, 6 Langley Street, Covent Garden, London WC2H 9JA.

World Health Organisation (1989) Protecting, promoting and supporting breast-feeding – the special role of the maternity services. A joint WHO/UNICEF Statement. WHO, Geneva.

■ Suggested further reading

Vallenas C, Savage F (1998) Evidence for the Ten Steps to Successful Breastfeeding. Division of Child Health and Development, WHO, Geneva.

Inch S, Fisher C (1998) Breastfeeding. In Marsh G, Renfrew M (eds) Community Based Maternity Care. Oxford, Oxford University Press, Chapter 24.

Becoming Baby Friendly – the video 1999 Mark-It TV. In press.

Chapter 6

Sexual health in the postnatal period

Jill Stewart-Moore

■ Introduction

Family planning has been seen as part of the midwife's role for almost three decades in the UK. In 1973, the World Health Organisation (WHO) proposed that family planning should be regarded as a regular and integral part of nursing and midwifery functions rather than a separate entity. A public health paper (WHO 1973) laid out the minimum requirements for nurse and midwife education programmes to include family planning, human reproduction and population dynamics. The paper foresaw that future generations of students would not require such detailed education as it would already have been accomplished through mass communication. Today, new dimensions to the challenge of sex education have emerged. The rise in the number of newly reported cases of human immunodeficiency virus (HIV) infection and the continuing high number of pregnancies to the under-16s demonstrates limitations in the effectiveness of current efforts and has led to shortfalls in the government reaching its targets for sexual health under the Health of the Nation strategy (Adler 1997).

The specialty of family planning is adapting its structure and scope. Greenhouse (1994) suggests that all services addressing the medical and psychological needs of sexually active adolescent and adult women should be set up under one roof. Contraception clinics, he argues, should offer screening for sexually transmitted infections such as chlamydia, with a limited range of on-site antibiotics dispensed free of charge. HIV education should be fully integrated into sexual health promotion. Stedman and Elstein (1995) observe that family planning and genitourinary medicine are both concerned with preventing the adverse consequences of sexual intercourse: unintended pregnancy and genital infection. Just as these two specialties are collaborating, it is time for midwives to embrace the dual challenge of giving contraceptive advice and advice to prevent sexually transmitted infection. The arguments put forward in this chapter challenge midwives to adapt their practice and help women to achieve safe, fulfilling sexual enjoyment after childbirth.

■ It is assumed that you are already aware of the following:

- The anatomy of the pelvic floor and related structures;
- The physiological changes accompanying the postnatal period;
- The advantages, disadvantages and efficacy of the main methods of contraception;
- And have some experience of discussing family planning issues with women;
- And have reflected on your own sexuality and acknowledge the past experiences that influence your personal sexuality.

■ Sexual health

Sexual health means more than contraception. It has been described by the WHO (1986) as:

- A capacity to enjoy and control sexual and reproductive behaviour in accordance with a social and personal ethic
- Freedom from psychological factors that inhibit sexual response and impair sexual relationships
- Freedom from organic disorders, diseases and deficiencies that interfere with sexual and reproductive functions.

This definition offers three components of sexual health that will be used to focus the discussion in this chapter. The implications of each will be examined from the perspective of midwifery practice in the postnatal period.

■ Enjoying and controlling sexual and reproductive behaviour

□ The acceptability of postpartum family planning advice and trends in contraceptive choice

Midwives offer contraceptive knowledge to enable women to control reproduction. Several factors affect the acceptability of this advice. For some women, a resumption of sexual intercourse is not planned for some time. For others, a discussion about intimate relations is not welcome when the genital area is sore and they are adjusting to new perceptions of sexuality following childbirth. For many women, however, the opportunity to discuss planning or preventing future pregnancies is most welcome.

The quality and acceptability of providing immediate postpartum family planning advice has been studied by Jarvis and Lewis (1996). A postal survey to assess the efficacy of contraceptive advice provided to recently delivered women on the postnatal wards was conducted in Wigan and Leigh NHS Trust. Responses were received from 122 (39.4 per cent) of the 310 women delivered in March 1994. Ninety-three per cent (114) of the respondents were using contraception; 79 per cent reported receiving advice on postnatal wards, 80 per cent expressing satisfaction with this. However, 18 per cent of women replied that they did not wish to discuss contraception immediately after childbirth. This represents a significant proportion of women whose reservations need to be identified and respected.

The puerperium is a time of role change. Adaptation will include developing new boundaries and patterns of couple identity in relation to sexual adjustment, individual gratification, social relationships and interpersonal communication (Raphael-Leff 1991). Sexual adjustment often involves a change of contraceptive method. This adaptation is a process that may well be different month by month after childbirth. One limitation of Jarvis and Lewis's study (1996) is that the questionnaire was sent out 6 months after delivery, by which time some of the earlier perceptions of postnatal care may well have been forgotten.

Trends reflect changes in contraceptive use, and the analysis by McEwan *et al* (1997) of data concerning contraceptive use over the past 20 years offers some insight into contraceptive choices today. Even in 1971, ways were found of asking sensitive questions (McEwan *et al* 1997). For example, unmarried respondents were not asked whether they were sexually active or not but were asked whether they saw themselves as being 'at risk' of unplanned pregnancy. A comparison of three population surveys (1970, 1975 and 1990–91) indicates a very marked increase in the prevalence of sterilisation, particularly of vasectomy. McEwan *et al* (1997) describe how the condom and pill predominate over other methods in all years, although there has been a decline in use of the withdrawal method. Over the 20 years covered by the comparative surveys, the increased experience of all women of all contraceptive methods is noted. If this trend continues, midwives can expect to be required to provide information to women on the wide range of methods available in order to facilitate choice. The authors comment that the aim of family planning services to make a choice available to women seems to have been achieved. The message for midwives is to ensure that women are informed, in depth, of all the choices on offer and not to assume that a previously tried and tested method will be chosen again, especially if the method resulted in the current unplanned pregnancy!

☐ The midwife's role in giving family planning advice, and its timing

Jarvis *et al* (1996) have reviewed midwives' participation in family planning services on postnatal wards. Ninety midwives working in hospital and the community in Wigan and Leigh NHS Trust were asked their views on the place and time of the provision of contraceptive services in the postnatal period; 74 per cent responded. Almost all midwives felt themselves to be the most suitable professionals to discuss contraception. However, the advice was limited to those methods about which they felt confident. Fifty-five per cent of the midwives felt confident discussing the IUCD and natural methods, while only 21 per cent felt confident discussing progesterone implants and only 24 per cent felt confident discussing the female condom. The authors argue that family planning advice is an underutilised aspect of the midwife's role and that there is a need for further training and regular updating for the service to be successful (Jarvis *et al* 1996). A minority, 37 per cent of midwives, considered the postnatal visit to the GP to be the most appropriate time for family planning advice. This is clearly too late for some women as ovulation may have already occurred and, if sexual activity has commenced, the woman may already be pregnant (Everett 1997).

There is evidence of the importance of information on contraception being given early in the postnatal period. Bolam *et al* (1998) report a randomised controlled trial of the timing of postpartum education of mothers in Nepal, one of the least developed countries of the world. The prevalence of contraceptive use generally is quoted as 23 per cent and there are high infant and maternal mortality rates. In their study, women who received health education on family planning immediately after birth or at birth and at 3 months later were significantly more likely to be using family planning at 6 months than were those receiving it only at 3 months after birth or not at all. The health educators were deliberately selected as being likely to gain the respect of mothers through their experience as midwives or community health workers, but they were also able to put mothers at ease during the education session. This is an important quality issue for all sexual health advisors.

☐ Social and personal ethics: the diversity of women's cultures

Are health professionals meeting the needs of ethnic minority women in Britain? Raleigh *et al* (1997) studied data from the General Household Surveys of 1991–95, relating to women aged 16–49, to explore rates of fertility and contraceptive use among different groups of women. Women were grouped into the three following categories – White, African and Caribbean, and Indian, Pakistani and Bangladeshi – in order to generate sufficient numbers for reliable statistical analysis. The authors calculated that fertility was highest among the Indian, Pakistani and Bangladeshi women, being more than double that of the white women at age 35 years and over. They proposed that language difficulties, lack of information and a preference for female doctors might contribute to lower uptake of sexual health care among this group of women, and therefore to higher rates of fertility. The use of condoms and the intrauterine device was higher among Indian, Pakistani and Bangladeshi women than in the other groups. The contraceptive choices of African and Caribbean women are similar to those of white women except for a low prevalence of vasectomy in ethnic minority groups generally.

Raleigh *et al* (1997) argue that the higher perinatal and infant mortality in the Indian, Pakistani and Bangladeshi group results from their high fertility, short birth intervals and late childbearing. They conclude that some women from ethnic minority groups have unmet family planning needs and suggest that while the lower contraceptive use might reflect the desire for a larger family size, it might also indicate differences in attitudes or access to family planning services.

Differences in attitudes are the subject of useful work by Bowes and Domokos (1996) and their colleagues. These authors argue that the voices of Glaswegian Pakistani Muslim women have been muted by both gender and race, and they report using research interviews as a means of raising women's voices. The research was conducted in such a way that the women were largely in control of the interview and were able to ensure that their full views were heard. Using a process of empowerment in the research interview permits the expression of views that may well challenge dominant values. For example, many of the women interviewed expressed an appreciation of long postnatal stays in hospital. This research may be an appropriate model for further research to gain a better understanding of the sexual health and other needs of women from a diversity of cultures.

Sociocultural attitudes affect the resumption of sexual enjoyment after childbirth. El-Tomi *et al* (1993) describe the sexual adjustment during pregnancy and after childbirth of 160 Muslim women in Kuwait. Traditionally, among Kuwaitis, there is a 40-day voluntary abstinence from sexual intercourse. The authors consider that the voluntary 6 weeks' abstinence should not be ignored in the study, yet they report that 95 per cent of women in the study had resumed sexual intercourse by 8 weeks. It is unclear from the discussion of their findings whether the resumption of sexual intercourse had occurred only in the 2 weeks following abstinence or whether abstinence was generally not practised.

These studies should prompt midwives to re-examine the service we offer for the extent to which it takes into account cultural diversity. The availability of leaflets in appropriate languages and the time taken to explore contraception with women with limited English language skills requires consideration. The midwife has to tread a delicate path between ensuring that the information is available to those who wish to receive it and respect for the woman's control of her reproductive abilities. Acute sensitivity to the individual woman's needs is required.

■ Freedom from psychological factors that inhibit sexual response and impair sexual relationships

It has been suggested that childbirth reduces sexual desire, activity and enjoyment for at least 1 year after delivery (Demyttenaere *et al* 1995). The authors reviewed several studies mainly published in the 1980s and argue for a biopsychosocial analysis of the many factors influencing women's psychosexual adaptation after childbirth. The following section reviews some of the current research examining the many variables affecting the complex and sensitive area of sexual response in the postnatal period. On the basis of research evidence, midwives may be able to prepare women better to anticipate changes in their sexuality, facilitate discussion about the changes they experience and direct women to special professional support if necessary.

☐ Tiredness

Fatigue is a factor dominant in the recent literature in association with problems related to intercourse after childbirth. Brown and Lumley (1998) studied 1336 women who responded to a state-wide survey in Victoria, Australia. Questionnaires were sent to women 6–7 months after childbirth. Sixty-nine per cent of respondents complained of tiredness, this being the most common health problem. Twenty-six per cent complained of sexual problems. The women were also asked about what issues they would have liked more help with: areas mentioned most frequently were emotional well-being, general health and recovery, and tiredness. Brown and Lumley (1998) suggest that specific invitations by health professionals, including midwives, to discuss tiredness may be necessary for women to feel free to talk about its effects and possible solutions.

Glazener (1997) also found that women who reported perineal pain, depression or tiredness experienced problems related to intercourse more often than those who did not. She received 1249 replies to a postal questionnaire concerning women's postnatal experience in hospital in Grampian, Scotland. Ninety per cent of this sample completed further questionnaires at 8 weeks postpartum. Half of the original respondents were contacted again when their infants were 12–18 months old to enquire about their experience thus far; 438 (86 per cent) responded. At 2 months, postpartum depression and tiredness were significantly related to a lack of interest in intercourse.

Both of these studies (Glazener 1997; Brown & Lumley 1998) report high levels of fatigue interfering with women's sex lives. In a subject review, Demyttenaere *et al* (1995) suggest that loss of sexual interest may be a sign of postpartum depression, which may be masked. Given the high incidence of postpartum depression, this possibility needs to be considered.

☐ Breastfeeding

Another factor prominent in Glazener's study (1997, p. 332) was the link between 'breastfeeding and disinterest in intercourse'. Women in this study were three times less likely to be interested in intercourse if they were breast-feeding. A further investigation of the coital frequency of breastfeeding women with that of women artificially feeding their infants would be useful. If a low frequency of coitus while breastfeeding is generally the case, breast-feeding women may well be happy to use barrier methods to protect against pregnancy in the postnatal period. Although barrier methods are generally less effective than hormonal methods, they may be sufficient for the breast-feeding woman who is less fertile.

An additional insight into the association between breastfeeding and sexual desire and activity is offered by a study from Australia by Forster *et al* (1994), who aimed to examine, prospectively and daily, the effects of breastfeeding on the psychology, sexuality and behaviour of healthy primiparous women 6 months or more postpartum. The setting for the study was well chosen as Australia achieves a high incidence of women breastfeeding (Palmer 1993). Women completed a daily diary for at least 8 weeks before and after the cessation of breastfeeding. There was a signifi-cant change in mood, fatigue, sexual feelings and frequency of sexual intercourse in the 4 weeks after weaning. Mood improved after 4 weeks of weaning, fatigue improved and sexual activity significantly increased. The authors argue that since fatigue affects libido, this reduction of fatigue following weaning may be responsible for the change in sexual feelings. In addition, the cessation of breastfeeding for many women in the study coincided with the return of the menses, indicating a return of fertility. This study suggests that there is a need to inform women to use a more effective method of contraception to prevent unwanted pregnancy after weaning.

■ Freedom from organic disorders, diseases and deficiencies that interfere with sexual and reproductive functions

☐ Dyspareunia

Freedom from diseases and deficiencies that interfere with sexual activity includes the physical recovery of the genital tract after childbirth. Dyspare-unia – difficult or painful intercourse – may result from incomplete recovery. Studies indicate this problem may be more common than has been realised, and although it often presents beyond the postnatal period, there are impli-cations for midwifery practice.

Johanson *et al* (1993) studied 413 women in North Staffordshire Maternity Hospital, 100 of whom had a normal delivery, and 313 of whom had a forceps or ventouse delivery. The women were recruited for inclusion in the trial at 24 hours post-delivery. Their perineum was assessed for the degree of trauma, and a questionnaire was sent out in the second year after childbirth. Sixty-one per cent of women responded to the follow-up questionnaire. Findings indicated an association between perineal injury and later dyspareunia. Thirty-five per cent of women with perineal injury experienced painful intercourse, compared with only 17 per cent of those with an intact perineum. A higher proportion of women in the instrumental delivery group had dyspareunia. Discomfort at 1 year also related to early discomfort: those women with a painful perineum at 24–48 hours after delivery were more likely to experience later pain.

Physiotherapists Hay-Smith and Mantle (1996), on the basis of findings from a survey they conducted, go as far as recommending that all women should be offered information about dyspareunia and the service provided for sufferers. They invited a sample of 342 women, all of whom had had normal deliveries and were booked under a single consultant, to participate in a study of difficulty with intercourse after childbirth. An anonymous questionnaire was sent to the 103 women who agreed to participate. Fifty-five per cent of those responding reported experiencing superficial dyspareunia after childbirth, reaching a measurement of less than 50 mm on the 100 mm severity of pain with intercourse scale used in the study. The authors acknowledge that respondents were older and of higher socioeconomic class than the average, and were therefore not representative. When women were asked about it, few women reported confiding problems with intercourse to doctors or other health professionals. Reasons given for not consulting a doctor were that the pain went or was expected to go away on its own.

There is evidence that midwives could pay particular attention to women at higher risk of postpartum morbidity by preparing them for the days ahead. By giving them permission to disclose issues in their sexual lives to professionals, midwives may give women the courage later to seek help for their sexual problems. Instrumental delivery and/or a painful perineum at 24–48 hours are predictors of later dyspareunia. These women in particular could be informed of the availability of local physiotherapist/gynaecologist service provision.

■ Screening for disease and sexually transmitted infection

The postnatal period has been commonly used as an opportunity for screening for a range of conditions of the genital tract. It is important to consider the effectiveness of such efforts as well as to link them to health promotion information for women.

☐ Cervical cancer

Guidelines produced by the NHS Cervical Screening Programme (NHSCSP) (Duncan 1997) challenge many of the practices previously incorporated into maternity care. In particular, additional cervical smears are not required in association with pregnancy provided that the woman has had a smear within the last 3–5 years, and teenagers are no longer targeted for screening.

Several studies have altered the view that adolescents engaging in unprotected sexual activity are a risk group for cervical cancer. Bloomfield and Duncan (1994), in a review of five studies of the incidence of cytological abnormality in teenagers, reported a low incidence of cervical intra-epithelial neoplasia grade III. The authors argue that there is no justification for the routine screening of teenagers if the lesion can be detected at a later date before invasion has occurred. Sankar and Tayal (1998), in an audit of 3377 smears in Newcastle upon Tyne, found that most of the abnormal smears in woman under 20 years of age were mild, and the frequency of significant premalignant cervical abnormality in teenagers was low.

The goal of the NHSCSP is to reduce mortality from cervical cancer, and reducing the number of unnecessary smears is important to improve the specificity and efficiency of the programme. Midwives assisting or performing cervical smears should heed these recommendations.

☐ Chlamydia

Data are emerging, as diagnostic techniques improve, that genital *Chlamydia trachomatis* is a cause of postpartum cervicitis and endometritis, resulting from organisms ascending mucosal surfaces (Ruby 1998). These organisms are often harboured asymptomatically in the vagina prior to delivery, having been transmitted by sexual intercourse. Other organisms, such as *Gardnerella vaginalis*, act in the same way, causing wound infection and puerperal sepsis (Woodrow & Lamont 1998).

When cultures of vaginal swabs reveal such infections postpartum, the midwife needs to ensure that the paediatric staff caring for the baby are informed and that the partner is also advised. Informing contacts of exposure to a sexually transmitted infection is usually the role of the genitourinary medicine department. Appropriate investigation and treatment may prevent the woman's reinfection. Ongoing untreated genital tract infection makes men and women more vulnerable to infection from HIV if they are exposed to it (Pratt 1995).

☐ Human immunodeficiency virus (HIV)

Midwives and obstetricians have recently come under fire for not broaching HIV testing in the antenatal period (Mercey 1998), in spite of Department of Health guidelines that recommend offering HIV testing to all pregnant women in high prevalence areas and to any woman who might have been exposed to infection (DoH 1992). Without the opportunity for antenatal diagnosis, women with HIV infection are effectively denied access to the increasing number of interventions to reduce the risk of infection to their babies and the possibility of early treatment for themselves. A number of initiatives have been developed to address this issue. Recommendations have been published to improve the uptake of antenatal HIV testing (Intercollegiate Working Party for Enhancing Voluntary Confidential HIV Testing in Pregnancy 1998), the Department of Health has issued a leaflet for women about antenatal HIV testing, to be used in areas of high prevalence for HIV, and the Royal College of Midwives has undertaken an educational campaign to support midwives in this effort.

It is also worth considering how HIV awareness could extend into the postnatal period, when messages about safer sex can be addressed. In New York, where HIV infection is strongly associated with drug use, HIV testing is discussed with women postnatally if they have not received counselling and testing antenatally. In a study in the Bronx, New York, 544 women were interviewed postnatally in a study of knowledge, attitudes and behaviours in relation to HIV, and the interview findings were considered in relation to selected variables from the women's notes (Webber *et al* 1997). Of particular concern were the women with a history of drug use, who were nine times as likely as others to report no prenatal care. Without antenatal HIV testing, these women, at increased risk of HIV, are unable to choose interventions to reduce the risk of transmission to their babies.

Similar findings about the low rate of antenatal diagnosis of HIV pertain in the UK. Ongoing surveys of HIV seroprevalence among pregnant women, considered in relation to reports of known cases of infection, indicate that only 10 per cent of previously undiagnosed pregnant women are diagnosed during pregnancy care (Nicoll *et al* 1998). Richardson and Sharland (1998) report that, in South London, since 1992 when the Department of Health guidelines on antenatal testing were first introduced (DoH 1992), only 1 in 17 cases of HIV-positive children were anticipated by antenatal testing. The median age of presentation of the disease in 24 children born after 1992 was 19 months. Mercey (1998) argues that, by this late stage, a subsequent pregnancy may well have already started.

Postnatal care offers an additional opportunity to discuss HIV infection and to offer testing and diagnosis.

☐ Female-controlled barriers: increased protection

Protection for women from sexually transmitted disease, including the human papilloma virus, one of the factors responsible for cervical cancer (Duncan 1997), is paramount in sexual health advice.

Commenting on 10 studies comparing the effects of condoms, diaphragms and spermicides on sexually transmitted disease prevention, Rosenberg and Gollub (1992) note that 9 out of the 10 studies found a lower risk of sexually transmitted disease among the users of female-controlled devices. The authors go on to argue that diaphragms and spermicides should receive greater emphasis in prevention messages; they are considerably safer than unprotected sex. Spermicide use is associated with a decreased incidence of cervical cancer (Rosenberg & Gollub 1992). The limitation of the diaphragm is that it leaves the vagina and vulva exposed to the penis and the ejaculate. However, the cervix is blocked from invasion by microorganisms such as chlamydia and the gonococci that usually enter via the cervix (Stein 1993). Cervical ectopy, the displacement of the cervical squamocolumnar junction distally, is common in oral contraceptive users. As ectopy increases women's susceptibility to HIV, Stein (1993) argues that the diaphragm offers protection to pill users. The 'belt and braces' approach, using the pill and condoms together, is commonly recommended and increasingly being taken up. The diaphragm and the pill offer wider scope to couples who cannot accept condom use. Observational studies indicate a 50–75 per cent effectiveness for the diaphragm as a barrier for cervical pathogens and an average 82 per cent contraceptive effectiveness (Rosenberg & Gollub 1992; Bounds 1994).

Owen and Caudill (1996) argue that current contraceptive clinical trials are conducted to find how well a method works in optimal circumstances, but what is missing is how the method works in the everyday lives of women, including intermittent or improper use. They observe that female medical practitioners are more likely than males to recommend the diaphragm to their clients and that client satisfaction is highest with female health care providers of contraception. The strength of the midwifery profession is that it is a predominantly female profession. Midwives are challenged to ensure that recommending diaphragm use is part of their regular family planning advice, particularly as part of a double package: a barrier to protect against disease with the pill or coil to prevent pregnancy.

An alternative female-controlled method is the female condom. Advantages include the strong material, polyurethane, that is less likely to rupture or to contain pinholes than the male condom. Couples may engage in sexual intercourse before full erection of the penis. The female condom covers both the internal and external genitalia, providing protection against sexually transmitted disease (Farr *et al* 1994). Existing research on the use of the female condom has limitations. These include small sample size (Gollub *et al* 1995) and the sampling having been restricted to women who had to use the device as their only means of contraception for 6 months (Farr *et al* 1994).

In an American study, Sly *et al* (1997) compared women who tried the device with those who did not, and characteristics and reactions to the device among women who used the female condom during at least half of their sexual encounters compared with less regular users of the method. Black and Hispanic women were more likely to use the female condom than were white women. Thirty-eight per cent of women who used the device for at least half of their sexual encounters were aged under 25. The data also suggest that women's satisfaction with the device increases as they use it more regularly. Difficulty with insertion and the device slipping during use were more likely to be reported in the study by less regular users. The contraceptive efficacy of the female condom is in the same range as other barrier methods (Sly *et al* 1997). To summarise, some women, apparently younger women, have a positive experience of female condom use. For others, the method interferes with or detracts from the sexual experience to an unacceptable degree (Sly *et al* 1997).

■ Sensitivity in giving sexual health advice

The midwife may feel it inappropriate to offer sexual health advice with family planning advice in a seemingly stable period of the women's life. A sensitive approach is required when suggesting the prevention of sexually transmitted disease as infidelity in the couple's relationship may be implied. However, the chances of the woman staying with the one partner in a lifetime are statistically low. Evidence from the government-initiated survey into sexual health in Great Britain (Wellings *et al* 1994) indicates that the average person reaching the age of 18 in the 1990s can expect to have 18 sexual partners in a lifetime. The study, using a questionnaire, face-to-face interview format for 18,876 people in Britain, revealed a pattern of increasing frequency of partner change with successive generations. The survey identifies those who are separated, divorced or widowed as having particularly rapid partner change. This group is five times as likely to report 'unsafe sex' as those who are married. Wellings *et al* (1994) suggest that they are a neglected audience in terms of health education intervention. The midwife is in a key position to give advice as many women may not talk about sexual health with any other health professional during the childbearing years. However, research has yet to be undertaken on the acceptability of such advice. It is interesting to note that it has taken until the 1990s for research to emerge on the acceptability of family planning advice in the postnatal period, let alone the acceptability of sexual health advice at that time.

From some midwives' viewpoints, the postnatal period, with all its emotional upheaval and uncertainty in the woman's life about accepting a newborn child, may be seen as an inappropriate time to talk about wider relationship issues, especially those which call for a change in relationship practice, such as introducing barrier methods of contraception. Some of these issues are addressed in work by Willig (1994) in her discourse analysis of 14 semi-structured interviews with couples about condom use. Accounts of condom use were analysed to obtain a better understanding of their use by heterosexual adults. The resulting discourse constructs marriage as a condition incompatible with condom use. There was an assumption among respondents that to raise the issue of condom use with one's partner might well constitute a serious threat to the integrity of the relationship itself as trust would be jeopardised. The continuation of trust meant not raising challenging questions. Willig's (1994) study contributes to our understanding of why both married and unmarried couples may be reluctant to request condom use by their partners.

Prochaska *et al*'s (1992) model of behaviour change suggests how people change. The modification of behaviours involves progression through five stages: precontemplation, contemplation, preparation, action and maintenance. Contemplation is the stage in which people are aware that a problem exists and are seriously thinking about overcoming it but have not yet made a commitment to take action. Change can be effected by an advancement of knowledge in the contemplative stage of the cycle, which is then acted on when the time is right. Condom use may not be introduced in the present relationship in the postnatal period, but if sexual relationships change or there is there is a further stimulus to change, the advice may then be remembered.

Sexual health education by the midwife in the postnatal period may not be acted on immediately but may produce later changes. Health professionals' reluctance to introduce the issue represents a lost opportunity. Pappenheim (1995) describes how calls to the Family Planning Association helpline illustrate that communication about sexual matters is fraught with ambiguity and inhibition.

Midwives can use their skills to break the national taboo of communicating about sex.

■ Recommendations for clinical practice in the light of currently available evidence

1. A small proportion of women will not want to discuss sex and contraception immediately after childbirth. Their wishes need to be respected.

2. Midwives need to be regularly updated on contraception and sexual health advice.

3. All women need to be informed that they may fall pregnant before their menstrual periods return and to take precautions to avoid unwanted pregnancy. Tact is needed when dealing with all women, and midwives should be sensitive to cultural perspectives other than their own.

4. Women should be informed of the risks of sexually transmitted disease, especially if they change partner or have several partners. Separated, divorced or widowed women are more likely to engage in unsafe sex. The value of wearing a condom to prevent disease as well as using another method to prevent pregnancy should be presented as the safest option. Include the option of the diaphragm if condoms are unacceptable. The 'belt and braces' method of the pill and condom or diaphragm is the safest option.

5. When a vaginal swab reveals sexually transmitted infection postpartum, the woman should be referred to the genitourinary medicine department. Confidential partner notification and treatment can be offered.

6. All newly delivered women should be made aware of local services for dyspareunia. Women who had an instrumental delivery or who have a sore perineum at 24–48 hours are more likely to suffer dyspareunia and especially need this information.

7. Women who are breastfeeding are likely to have a lower incidence of coitus, and barrier methods of contraception may be sufficient. After weaning, a more effective method of contraception may be necessary to prevent unwanted pregnancy.

8. In areas of high HIV prevalence, a postpartum discussion of HIV testing may be considered for women who have not been involved in such an exchange antenatally.

9. Cervical smear tests are not indicated just because the women have been pregnant provided that the woman has had a smear in the past 3–5 years. Teenagers need not be included in the cervical screening programme.

10. Auditing service users' perceptions of sexual health advice in the postnatal period should be considered. Gaining feedback from women in ethnic minority communities, perhaps through link workers if there are language barriers, should be part of this effort.

■ Practice check

● Before starting to introduce sexual health issues, do you always confirm that the conversation is confidential?

● What steps do you take to put the woman at ease before discussing sex?

● What tips on the resumption of sexual intercourse do you include when discussing family planning? For example:

  – Encouraging pelvic floor exercises to increase vaginal tone;

  – The use of water-based lubricants (KY Jelly), particularly for breast-feeding mothers;

  – Warning breastfeeding mothers that their breasts may leak at orgasm;

  – Suggesting controlled male penetration. Kitzinger (1994) gives further guidance and pictures of comfortable positions for love-making after childbirth.

● Where are your local family planning clinics? Are there specialist sessions for teenagers?

● The under-16s require special consideration in relation to sexual health care. They should be advised to tell their parents that they are seeking such advice and treatment. Belfield (1997) explains further the legal and ethical issues surrounding sexual health advice to under-16-year-olds.

● What is the availability of sterilisation services in your local hospital? Is vasectomy only available privately? What are the waiting lists for male and female sterilisation?

● Are you up to date on the newer methods of contraception such as implants and the female condom?

● Is contraceptive information available in the languages of the local population?

● Do you know the women link workers working with local minority ethnic groups? Are there special cultural taboos surrounding sex in the postnatal period?

■ References

Adler MA (1997) Sexual health – a health of the nation failure. British Medical Journal, 314: 1743–7.

Belfield T (1997) FPA Contraceptive Handbook, 2nd edn. Family Planning Association, London.

Bloomfield PI, Duncan ID (1994) Cervical screening and teenage women. In Bonnar J (ed.) Recent Advances in Obstetrics and Gynaecology. Churchill Livingstone, Edinburgh, pp. 155–60.

Bolam A, Manandhar DS, Shresha P, Ellis M, Costello de LAM (1998) The effects of postnatal education for mothers on infant care and family planning practices in Nepal: a randomised controlled trial. British Medical Journal, 316: 805–11.

Bounds W (1994) Contraceptive efficacy of the diaphragm and cervical caps used in conjunction with spermicide: a fresh look at the evidence. British Journal of Family Planning, 20: 84–7.

Bowes AM, Domokos TM (1996) Pakistani women and maternity care: raising muted voices. Sociology of Health and Illness, 18(1): 45–65.

Brown S, Lumley J (1998) Maternal health after childbirth: results of an Australian population based survey. British Journal of Obstetrics and Gynaecology, 105: 156–61.

Demyttenaere K, Gheldof M, Van Assche FA (1995) Sexuality in the postpartum period: a review. Current Obstetrics and Gynaecology, 5: 81–4.

Department of Health (1992) Guidelines for Offering Voluntary Named HIV Antibody Testing to Women Receiving Antenatal Care. DoH, London.

Duncan I (ed.) (1997) Guidelines for Clinical Practice and Programme Management, 2nd edn. National Health Service Screening Programme, Sheffield.

El-Tomi NF, Al Bustan M, Abokhadour N (1993) Maternal sexuality during pregnancy and after childbirth in Kuwait. International Quarterly of Community Health Education, 13(2): 163–73.

Everett S (1997) Contraception. In Andrew G (ed.) Women's Sexual Health. Baillière Tindall, London, pp. 173–217.

Farr G, Gabelnick H, Sturgen K, Dorflinger L (1994) Contraceptive efficacy and acceptability of female condom. American Journal of Public Health, 84: 1960–4.

Forster C, Abraham S, Taylor A, Llewellyn-Jones D (1994) Psychological and sexual changes after the cessation of breast feeding. Obstetrics and Gynaecology, 84(5): 872–6.

Glazener CMA (1997) Sexual function after childbirth: women's experiences, persistent morbidity and lack of professional recognition. British Journal of Obstetrics and Gynaecology, 104: 330–5.

Gollub EL, Stein Z, El–Sadr W (1995) Short term acceptability of the female condom among staff and patients at a New York City Hospital. Family Planning Perspectives, 27: 155–8.

Greenhouse P (1994) Under one roof: setting up sexual health services for women. Maternal and Child Health, (Jul): 228–33.

Hay-Smith J, Mantle J (1996) Surveys of the experience and perceptions of postnatal dyspareunia of post-natal women, general practitioners and physiotherapists. Physiotherapy, 82(2): 91–7.

Intercollegiate Working Party for Enhancing Voluntary Confidential HIV Testing in Pregnancy (1998) Reducing Mother to Child Transmission of HIV Infection in the United Kingdom. Royal College of Paediatrics and Child Health, London.

Jarvis RR, Lewis PA (1996) A survey of the quality and acceptability of immediate family planning advice in a hospital setting. British Journal of Family Planning, 22: 95–6.

Jarvis R, Lewis P, Blanchard S (1996b) Postnatal contraceptive advice: midwives' attitudes. British Journal of Family Planning, 22: 181–2.

Johanson R, Wilkinson P, Bastible A, Ryan S, Murphy H, O'Brien S (1993) Health after childbirth: a comparison of normal and assisted delivery. Midwifery, 9: 161–8.

Kitzinger S (1994) The Year After Childbirth. Oxford University Press, Oxford.

McEwan J, Wadsworth J, Johnson A, Wellings K, Field J (1997) Changes in the use of contraceptive methods in England and Wales over two decades: Margaret Bones' surveys and the National Survey of Sexual Attitudes and Lifestyles. British Journal of Family Planning, 23: 5–8.

Mercey D (1998) Antenatal HIV testing. British Medical Journal, 316: 241–2.

Nicoll A, McGarrigle C, Brady AR *et al* (1998) Epidemiology and detection of HIV-1 among pregnant women in the UK: results from national surveillance 1988–96. British Medical Journal, 316: 353–8.

Owen SA, Caudill SA (1996) Contraception and clinical science: the place of women in reproductive technology. In Parrott RL, Condit CM (eds) Evaluating Women's Health Messages. Sage, Thousand Oaks, CA, pp. 81–94.

Palmer G (1993) Who helps health professionals with breast-feeding? Midwives Chronicle and Nursing Notes, (May): 147–56.

Pappenheim K (1995) Sex: a national taboo. Midwives 108(1286): 70.

Pratt R (1995) HIV and AIDS: A Strategy for Nursing Care, 4th edn. Edward Arnold, London.

Prochaska JO, Di Clemente C, Norcross JC (1992) In search of how people change. American Psychologist, 47: 1102–14.

Raleigh S, Almond C, Kiri V (1997) Fertility and contraception among ethnic minority women in Great Britain. Health Trends, 29(4): 109–13.

Raphael-Leff J (1991) Psychological Processes of Childbearing. Chapman & Hall, London.

Richardson M, Sharland M (1998) Late diagnosis of paediatric HIV infection in south west London. British Medical Journal, 316: 271–2.

Rosenberg M, Gollub E (1992) Commentary: methods women can use that may prevent sexually transmitted disease, including HIV. American Journal of Public Health, 82(11): 1473–8.

Ruby C (1998) *Chlamydia trachomatis*: the issues for women and midwifery. MIDIRS Midwifery Digest 8(1): 42–3.

Sankar K, Tayal S (1998) Cervical smear: is screening of teenagers justified? International Journal of STD and AIDS, 9: 303.

Sly DF, Quadagno D, Harrison DF, Eberstein IW, Richman K, Bailey M (1997) Use of the female condom. Family Planning Perspectives, 2: 181–4.

Stedman Y, Elstein M (1995) Rethinking sexual health clinics. British Medical Journal, 310: 341–2.

Stein Z (1993) HIV Prevention: an update on the status of methods women can use. American Journal of Public Health, 83(10): 1379–81.

Webber MP, Schoenbaum EE, Banuck KA (1997) Correlates of voluntary immunodeficiency virus antibody testing reported by postpartum women. Journal of American Medical Women's Association, 52(2): 89–92.

Wellings K, Field J, Johnson AM, Wadsworth J (1994) Sexual Behaviour in Britain: The National Survey of Sexual Attitudes and Lifestyles. Penguin, London.

Willig C (1994) Marital discourse and condom use. In Aggleton P, Davies P, Hart G (eds) AIDS Foundations for the Future. Taylor & Francis, London.

Woodrow N, Lamont R (1998) Bacterial vaginosis: its importance in obstetrics. Hospital Medicine, 59(6): 447, 450.

World Health Organisation (1973) Family planning in the education of nurses and midwives. WHO, Geneva.

World Health Organisation (1986) Concepts for Sexual Health. EUR/ICP/MCH 521. WHO, Copenhagen.

■ Suggested further reading

Andrew G (ed.) (1997) Women's sexual health. Baillière Tindall, London.

Everett S (1998) Contraception and family planning. Baillière Tindall, London.

Chapter 7

Domestic violence and pregnancy: a midwifery issue

Chris Bewley and Andy Gibbs

■ Introduction

Domestic violence, sometimes called domestic abuse, can affect all members or ex-members of a family and can occur in same-sex relationships (Stanko 1997). Abuse can be physical, emotional, psychological or sexual and profoundly affects the everyday lives of many people, predominantly women and children. This chapter examines the nature and effects of abuse on individuals and on society, and includes research into the perpetrators of domestic violence. The effects of abuse on pregnant women and on children are discussed, together with their professional significance for midwives. Finally, suggestions are made for effective midwifery interventions using an interdisciplinary approach.

■ It is assumed that you are already aware of the following:

- The UKCC guidelines on *The Scope of Professional Practice* (UKCC 1992);

- The UKCC guidelines on confidentiality (UKCC 1996);

- The mechanism in your own area for responding to child protection issues;

- The Royal College of Midwives position paper on domestic abuse (RCM 1998).

■ Prevalence and nature of domestic violence

As previously stated, any family member can be abused. While the variety of factors offered to explain violence is diverse, Harwin (1997) suggests that the single common factor is the need for the abuser to control the abused person. Abuse may be of children, elders, same-sex sexual partners or the male partner being abused by the female, but by far the most common in prevalence and severity is the abuse of a woman by the man with whom she is having, or has in the past had, a sexual relationship (Bewley & Gibbs 1991).

Mooney's (1993) survey of the nature and prevalence of domestic violence across a wide social range in North London revealed that 29 per cent of the women studied had experienced physical abuse and 39 per cent emotional or physical abuse. Twenty-three per cent of the women had also been sexually abused.

The Women's Aid Federation of England (Harwin 1997) documents a wide range of physical, emotional and sexual abuse described by women seeking their help. Women's reports of physical violence include being punched, slapped, kicked, choked, stabbed and burnt. Psychological abuse includes being made to clean an already clean house, being isolated from friends and family, not being allowed to raise one's eyes from the pavement when walking, constantly being told how ugly or useless they are and being threatened with physical abuse. The man may also threaten to take the children away or harm them, and may break things that are important to the woman. Sexual abuse involves forced sex, degrading sexual practices or withholding sex in a way that makes the woman feel humiliated.

For women who are abused, home is not a secure place to be (Kent 1987). Statistics show overwhelming evidence that more females are killed by their partners or ex-partners than by strangers. The organisation Victim Support suggests that 42 per cent of all female homicides are perpetrated by male partners, as compared with 6 per cent of male homicides in which the woman murders her partner (Victim Support 1992). Approximately 100 women in England and Wales are murdered every year by a partner or ex-partner (Home Office 1996), and women are most vulnerable when they leave the relationship.

■ Perpetrators of domestic violence

The majority of work on the subject of domestic violence centres on female victims or survivors of violence and their coping mechanisms. At the margins of the issue are those who claim that there may well be a hidden issue of female violence towards males within domestic situations. It may be claimed that similar factors such as guilt and shame contribute to the non-reporting of violence. If anything, it is argued, the pressure on males to remain silent is greater as a consequence of gender stereotyping. At present, however, the consensus in the UK suggests that most domestic violence consists of violence inflicted on women by men. This is reflected in crime surveys indicating that 11.4 per cent of women and 4.5 per cent of men have been the victims of domestic violence (Scottish Office 1998).

In the US, there is disagreement on this issue (Kingston & Penhale 1995). Stanko (1997) identifies that, according to US surveys, wives hit their husbands slightly more often than husbands hit their wives. However, when the severity of the violence is considered, males are overwhelmingly more destructive in their attacks. It is suggested that because of the greater physical, financial and emotional injury suffered, women are the predominant victims. Overall, there is little evidence to suggest that women pose the same danger to men that men do to women.

The 1996 Scottish Crime Survey (Scottish Office 1998) revealed that women were twice as likely to have been threatened and also to have had force used against them by a partner. Women were also three times more likely than men to be choked, strangled, suffocated or forced to have sex, while the most common form of assault on men was having objects thrown at them.

The acknowledgment of domestic violence and abuse as a serious social issue has taken place only within the past 50 years. Prior to this, violence against women was actively condoned by the church and state under a patriarchal system sanctioning male domination and the subordination of women to men. Women were seen to be responsible for housekeeping, childcare and providing sexual relief for their male partners, while being absolutely faithful to them (Dobash & Dobash 1987). Failure to carry out these duties constituted grounds for criticism, punishment or correction. These views were (and still are in many cases) held by both men and women in society, women being seen as legitimate targets for punishment. Mooney's (1993) North London domestic violence survey included a group of some 500 men who were given various scenarios and asked whether they would use violence to resolve any of them. Only 37 per cent said that they would not respond violently. Yearnshire (1997) conducted research in the UK with 23 men in police custody following arrest at a domestic incident. Over half of these men showed a lack of awareness that their violent behaviour was criminal.

The premise that domestic abuse is a gender issue is not widely accepted. Women are more likely to be the victims of violence perpetrated by partners or ex-partners, while violent attacks against men are more often perpetrated by other men (Home Office 1996). In fact, the contribution of women to violent crime is very low. Those who are violent are likely to be so against their already violent husbands, children in their care or themselves, and there are major differences in the violence that men experience that differentiates it substantially from that experienced by women (Economic and Social Research Council 1998). Unlike women, men do not live in constant terror after separation, are rarely killed by women pursuing them and do not live in the climate of sexual terrorism that many women describe. A critical factor in determining the types of intervention made with violent men is the analysis of the nature of violence. These interventions are also mediated by the way in which domestic abuse is explained and understood (Economic and Social Research Council 1998).

There are many and varied explanations of domestic violence, which are reviewed by Mezey (1997). Physiological theories argue that certain genetic and physiological traits predispose all men to violence. The psychopathological perspectives suggest that the perpetrators are jealous and weak men. Other social learning theories suggest that violence is transmitted generationally. Finally, there are sociostructural theories that focus on factors such as economic conditions, relative poverty and poor job opportunities (Mezey 1997). It is important to note that just as there is no universally understood definition of domestic abuse, there is similarly no commonly agreed explanation of its causes. This lack of agreement is often a barrier to the application of interventions.

While campaigns such as Zero Tolerance stress that all men have the capacity to abuse, there have been limited attempts to identify the characteristics of perpetrators. Mezey (1997) reviews research evidence in this field. The review warns against attempting strict categorisation. Research either identifies personality types, such as that of Langley & Levy (1977), that suggest that abusers are alcoholics, psychotics, psychopaths and bullies, or describes the *modus operandi* as in the work of Simpson-Subotnik (1983). Langley and Levy (1977) and Simpson-Subotnik (1983) identified the overcontrolled and the undercontrolled batterer. The overcontrolled batterer is represented by an uncharacteristic explosion of anger followed by considerable guilt and remorse. This contrasts with the undercontrolled batterer who is unable to tolerate frustration and whose violence is repetitive and compulsive. Mezey (1997: 42) concludes that 'Men who batter their partners are not, in general, mentally ill, but have a range of personality deficits which centre around insecurity, inadequacy and dependency.' While these findings may be illuminating, they do not translate easily into practical application for health care professionals.

☐ Interventions with violent and abusive men

Identifying batterers, applying legal sanctions in an effective way, offering re-education programmes and condemning the use of violence within relationships may ultimately offer some protection and hope for victims.

There is some conflict regarding the resourcing of interventions with regard to violent men. Lloyd (1995) points out that, on one hand, there is the possibility of men's behaviour being changed as a result of treatment programmes forcing them to confront their violent behaviour, while on the other this raises the question of resources. The establishment of programmes for violent men may detract resources from the existing, if somewhat limited, support currently directed towards women who are experiencing violence. Hoyle (1998) argues that it is naïve to see the question of resources as an either/or issue, pointing out that both women and men would benefit from some forms of intervention and that successful programmes for men would ultimately help women.

Lloyd (1995) reviews a range of social work interventions and highlights difficulties in identifying the most appropriate form of intervention with men, suggesting that there are potential dilemmas to be faced at each stage of intervention. For example, while arrest and prosecution are shown to produce a reduction or cessation in violence, they may also increase women's vulnerability. Additionally, schemes in Scotland whereby men were diverted from prosecution into conciliation and reparation schemes attracted criticism and strong objections from Scottish Women's Aid, who pointed out that such a strategy could imply that domestic violence was not an issue worthy of legal sanction. Reconsideration of the policy has led to intervention programmes being provided after the case has gone to court. Similarly, interventions such as family therapy and couple therapy may suggest that domestic violence is a consequence of family interactions and therefore a family problem, rather than challenging and focusing on the man's violent behaviour. This is also questioned as recent research suggests that women victims prefer not to involve the criminal justice system (Hoyle 1998).

Contemporary interventions such as the CHANGE programme based at Stirling University establish mechanisms whereby the offender is the joint responsibility of the courts and social work (Johnson 1995). A systematic programme confronts and challenges the man's violent behaviour, seeking for him to accept responsibility for his actions and to establish alternative ways of responding within relationships.

Whatever approaches are adopted to deal with violent men, the effects of violent behaviour on pregnant women have direct consequences on the pregnancy, as the next section shows.

■ Effects of abuse on pregnancy

Gelles (1975) was one of the first researchers into family violence to detect a link between pregnancy and the beginning or escalation of abuse. Other researchers (Dobash & Dobash 1987) noted that triggers for arguments and violence in relationships focused on money, housework, sexual services and excessive jealousy or possessiveness on the man's part. In pregnancy, those three areas of potential conflict are all affected (Bewley & Gibbs 1991). The birth of a child carries financial implications. Women, especially in early pregnancy, are tired and may experience diminished libido. The fetus may be a target for jealousy since it occupies the woman's body, which the man has previously considered available solely for his use. Abuse during pregnancy can lead to preterm labour, low birthweight babies, placental abruption, chorioamnionitis and actual fetal injury to limbs and organs (Bohn 1990; Norton *et al* 1995). Mooney (1993) showed that women who are abused are three times more likely to experience miscarriage. Edwards (1997) quotes two cases in which pregnant women were stabbed or kicked, resulting in death to the fetus from direct injury. Death was caused in one case by intracranial haemorrhage, and in the other by prematurity and stab wounds.

Blows to the pregnant abdomen can cause the release of arachidonic acid from damaged tissues. Arachidonic acid is a precursor of prostaglandins, which lead to uterine contractions and possible miscarriage or preterm labour. Research suggests that, during pregnancy, the focus of physical violence changes and that attacks are more likely to be targeted at the breasts, abdomen and genitals, almost a direct attack on the fetus (Bohn 1990; Berenson *et al* 1994).

The above examples are of physical violence, but stress associated with all types of abuse may lead the woman to use alcohol, drugs or cigarettes in an effort to make her life more tolerable. These all have well-documented adverse effects on both mother and baby. Additionally, stress has physical effects in the form of raising adrenaline levels, diverting blood from vital centres and reducing placental perfusion (Newton & Hunt 1984). Abused women show a higher rate of psychiatric illness, depression and suicide attempts (Mezey 1997) and may be more prone to postnatal depression.

■ Recognising abuse

It is suggested that adverse pregnancy outcome related to abuse is more common than placenta praevia and gestational diabetes, two conditions for which we routinely offer screening (Bohn 1990). Midwives belong to a profession that serves pregnant women so the detection of abuse is important in the care they give. However, women who are abused deserve help in their own right rather than only when their pregnancy is deemed to be affected. Their entire lives and those of their children are affected by abuse and the threat of abuse.

Since almost all pregnant women will have some form of contact with health professionals during or after pregnancy, it is vital that what McFarlane et al (1992) call a 'window of opportunity' to help an abused woman is not lost. Recognition and appropriate information and referral may enable an abused woman to rethink her position and seek help.

Women who are abused do not conform to a particular stereotype. They come from all socioeconomic groups and from all cultures, and in many cases there will be little indication of their abuse. There are, however, certain indicators that may lead midwives to believe that a women is being abused and needs an opportunity to talk (Helton 1987). Indicators may include:

- Obvious injuries, old bruises or burn marks, and injuries that are inconsistent with the woman's explanation of how they occurred;

- Smoking, alcohol or drug abuse;

- A past history of miscarriage, preterm labour and/or low birthweight babies;

- Frequent complaints of vaginal discharge, vaginal infection, pelvic pain or urinary tract infections;

- Difficulty sleeping, signs of depression or attempted suicide.

As well as physical signs, the woman and/or her partner may also behave in a way indicating the possibility of abuse:

- Making excuses for the partner, for example, 'He's got a terrible temper, but he's marvellous with the children';

- The partner threatening or frightening her, possibly being excessively jealous;

- The partner continually making disparaging remarks about her;

- The partner breaking things that belong to the woman;

- The partner staying close to the woman all the time to prevent her telling anyone what is happening.

This is not, however, an exhaustive list. On many occasions, midwives may feel that something is just not right, and if this is the case, they should act on their instincts and ask the woman, in private, about her circumstances (Bewley & Gibbs 1991). Contrary to popular belief, women express relief if they are given an opportunity to talk about their situation (Johnson 1995). Abused women cite many instances of visiting their GP or presenting at the accident and emergency unit with severe injuries (Johnson 1995), and of staff accepting their explanations of how they were injured, even when it was patently obvious that the injury could not have been caused in the way they described. By acting in this way, staff collude to keep abuse hidden and compound the myth that what goes on between couples in their own home is private and that no one should interfere (Bewley & Gibbs 1994).

■ Asking sensitive questions

Research in Tayside (Tayside Women and Violence Working Group 1994) revealed that health professionals cited embarrassment and not knowing what to say as significant reasons for non-intervention even when they felt sure that women were being abused. In many states in the USA and Canada, women who present for any form of health care are routinely asked about domestic abuse. A comparison between levels of disclosure of abuse by Norton *et al* (1995) revealed that women are most likely to talk about their abuse if they are given a questionnaire and guided through it by someone trained in its use. This type of screening would be difficult to implement in the UK since screening can only be carried out in situations where there is good multiagency provision of support for abused women. It would be unethical to encourage disclosure in the absence of a sound supportive infrastructure and system for referral. Although it has the advantage of allowing women who exhibit no signs of abuse to disclose their situation, a disadvantage of such screening is that it concentrates mainly on physical abuse, which may be episodic, whereas emotional abuse affects every moment of the woman's life yet may not be detected by such screening.

Nevertheless, it is important to recognise that there are some basic steps that can be taken to help abused women even where support systems are not available. Sensitive questioning, and the giving of appropriate information, signal to the woman that she is believed and not judged as being weak and foolish for remaining in an abusive situation. Education programmes for staff improve their ability to identify and communicate with abused women and help women to formulate strategies for remaining in a relationship or escaping from it (Helton 1987; Young & McFarlane 1991; Mandt 1993).

A number of agencies, including the Royal College of Midwives (RCM, 1998), have now issued guidelines that include examples of how to broach the subject. Although the guidelines vary between organisations, they all advocate a multiagency approach, which offers consistent advice and collaboration to ensure that women receive appropriate information and support. They also stress the importance of privacy and the need for any discussions to take place away from the partner. The questions below appear in one form or another in most of the professional guidelines, including those of the Royal College of Midwives (RCM 1998).

General questions that invite the woman to talk include:

- Is everything all right at home?

- Is anyone hurting you at home?

- Are you frightened of anyone at home?

- Does your partner break things that belong to you?

More specific questions or statements are:

- I notice you have some bruising. Did anyone at home do that to you?

- Some women tell me that their partners hit them. Has that happened to you?

■ Formulating local guidelines

Professional guidelines are extremely useful because they signal to members of the profession that they are supported by their professional body. A small unpublished survey of midwives by Tucker (1995) suggested that midwives need guidelines that are supportive but not prescriptive, and whose implementation is not mandatory. Local guidelines need to take account of what services are available for abused women and to consider women with special needs such as those who are disabled, those in same-sex relationships and those who have particular cultural needs.

In most areas, there is a domestic violence forum set up to improve communication between the various agencies who come into contact with abused women. This group consists of representatives from police domestic violence units, GPs, health visitors, Women's Aid, Alcoholics Anonymous, social services and so on, details usually being available from local town halls. Within domestic violence forums, multiagency strategies for the provision of information and referral can be formulated that fully involve the woman as prime decision-maker. However, midwives are not often represented in these groups, which is ironic, given the increasing evidence presented within this chapter that pregnant and newly delivered women may be at increased risk of violence.

While the existence of committees provides a good starting point, the primary factor in effective support comes from co-operation at 'grass-roots' level. Practitioners should be encouraged to consult colleagues in other professions and not make assumptions about what another professional group's role and responsibilities are.

■ Domestic abuse and child protection

Maintaining confidentiality on behalf of a client can raise issues of conflicting loyalties for the midwife. Midwives strive to keep what women tell them confidential, yet there are occasions on which it may be in the woman's best interests to disclose her situation to other members of the health care team. Research suggests that between 27 and 70 per cent of men who abuse their partners will also abuse their children (NCH Action for Children 1994; Johnson 1995). Where child abuse is suspected, the midwife has a statutory duty of disclosure (UKCC 1996) and must know how to implement child protection initiatives. The midwives in Tucker's (1995) study feared that intervention in suspected child abuse would result in children being summarily removed from their homes. However, as Fraser (1997) shows, raising concerns about abuse sets in motion a process in which parents are kept fully involved and informed while maintaining the safety of the child. The decision to remove a child is taken only in extreme circumstances; where the mother is not the abuser, the emphasis is on supporting her and the children while taking steps to exclude the abusing partner (Harwin 1997).

Even where children are not physically abused themselves they often witness or overhear the abuse of their mother, which can have longlasting psychological consequences for them (Harwin 1997). However, there is no concrete evidence to support the view that children brought up in abusive homes either go on to become abusers themselves or to be attracted into abusive relationships (Stanko 1997).

■ Keeping midwives safe

Midwives operate in premises and visit areas that may place them at risk of violence. Tucker's (1995) study showed that midwives feared for their own safety where they knew of a situation in which a male partner was violent. Midwives have a right to go about their work without fear of being molested, and many Trusts take the issue of staff safety very seriously. When faced with a violent situation, midwives should call for hospital security or the police. In extreme cases, midwives are entitled to withdraw their services if they feel threatened (UKCC 1996). However there are some additional steps that can be taken to maximise safety, especially in the community. The provision of mobile telephones and personal alarms can help to ensure safety, and midwives should ensure that their whereabouts and the time when they are expected back at base are known. Midwives should not travel alone to homes where there is a perceived threat of violence. Staff should also be trained in conflict avoidance in order to prevent aggressive situations escalating into violence (Bewley & Gibbs 1997).

■ Conclusion

Domestic abuse is a matter of social concern and public health. While recognising that it is a complex issue, it is not one that midwives can fail to engage with as doing so may collude with or perpetuate violence against women. There are actions and interventions that midwives may take at individual, local and national levels, some of which would be easy to implement. However, it is important that intervention is made from an informed perspective that maintains the autonomy of the woman.

■ Recommendations for clinical practice in the light of currently available evidence

Given the clear indications that violence is often directed against pregnant women, the following list provides a starting point for appropriate midwifery intervention.

1. The availability of local support and information should be prominently advertised by means of posters from Women's Aid, the police domestic violence unit, the local men's support group and so on.

2. Information and telephone numbers need to be included in information booklets about hospital/clinic services for pregnant women.

3. Posters showing relevant telephone numbers, and tear-off pads on which they can be written without this being seen to be done, can be made available in female toilets.

4. There should be ongoing, multiprofessional education for staff in relation to the prevalence and effects of domestic abuse.

5. Clear local guidelines for discussion and referral should exist.

6. Midwives must be involved in the multiagency approach to care.

7. The observation of overattentive partners who may be reluctant to leave women alone and/or who behave in ways that are disparaging to the woman is important.

8. Privacy must be provided.

9. There should be a means of documenting information where it cannot be seen by the partner.

■ Practice check

● Examine your own views on midwives' involvement in helping abused women.

● Have you come across women who you know or suspect were being abused but whom you did not know how to help? What would you do differently now?

● Check your own clinic and work area for posters and information on help for abused women and children.

● Review your Trust's policy on keeping employees safe. Are notices prominently displayed to state the Trust's policy on violence against its staff?

■ References

Berenson AB, Weimann CM, Wilkinson GS, Jones WA, Anderson GD (1994) Perinatal morbidity associated with violence experienced by pregnant women. American Journal of Obstetrics and Gynecology, 170: 1760–9.

Bewley CA, Gibbs A (1991) Violence in pregnancy. Midwifery, 7: 107–12.

Bewley CA, Gibbs A (1994) Coping with domestic violence in pregnancy. Nursing Standard, 8: 25–8.

Bewley CA, Gibbs A (1997) The role of the midwife. In Bewley S, Friend J, Mezey G (eds) Violence Against Women. RCOG Press, London, pp. 199–210.

Bohn DK (1990) Domestic violence in pregnancy: implications for practice. Journal of Nurse Midwifery, 35: 86–98.

Dobash R, Dobash R (1987) Violence towards wives. In Orford J (ed.) Coping with Disorder in the Family. Croom Helm, London, pp. 169–81.

Economic and Social Research Council (1998) Taking Stock; What do we Know about Violence. Economic and Social Research Council, Swindon.

Edwards S (1997) The law and domestic violence. In Bewley S, Friend J, Mezey G (eds) Violence Against Women. RCOG Press, London, pp 89–107.

Fraser J (1997) Child Protection: A Guide for Midwives. Books for Midwives Press, Hale.

Gelles R (1975) Violence and pregnancy; a note on the extent of the problem and needed services. Family Co–ordinator, 24: 816.

Harwin N (1997) Understanding women's experience of abuse. In Bewley S, Friend J, Mezey G (eds) Violence Against Women. RCOG Press, London, pp. 59–75.

Helton A (1987) A Protocol of Care for the Battered Woman. March of Dimes Birth Defects Federation, New York.

Home Office (1996) Criminal Statistics for England and Wales. HMSO, London.

Hoyle C (1998) Negotiating Domestic Violence: Police, Criminal Justice and Victims. Open University Press, Milton Keynes.

Johnson N (1995) Domestic violence: an overview. In Kingston P, Penhale B (eds) Family Violence and the Caring Professions. Macmillan, Basingstoke, pp. 1–26.

Kent A (1987) Home is where the fear is. Nursing Times, 85: 16–17.

Kingston P, Penhale B (1995) Family Violence and the Caring Professions. Macmillan, Basingstoke.

Langley R, Levy RC (1977) Wife Beating: The Silent Crisis. EP Dutton, New York.

Lloyd S (1995) Social work and domestic violence. In Kingston P, Penhale B (eds) Family Violence and the Caring Professions. Macmillan, Basingstoke, pp. 149–77.

McFarlane J, Parker B, Soeken K, Bullock L (1992) Assessing for abuse during pregnancy. Journal of the American Medical Association, 267: 3176–8.

Mandt A (1993) The curriculum revolution in action: nursing and crisis intervention for victims of family violence. Journal of Nurse Education, 32: 44–6.

Mezey G (1997) Perpetrators of domestic violence. In Bewley S, Friend J, Mezey G (eds) Violence Against Women. RCOG Press, London, pp. 35–44.

Mooney J (1993) The Hidden Figure: The North London Domestic Violence Survey. Middlesex University Centre for Criminology, London.

NCH Action for Children (1994) The Hidden Victims: Children and Domestic Violence. NCH Action for Children, London.

Newton RW, Hunt LP (1984) Psychosocial stress in pregnancy and its relation to low birth weight. British Medical Journal, 288: 1191–4.

Norton LB, Peipart JF, Zierler S (1995) Battering in pregnancy: an assessment of two screening methods. Obstetrics and Gynecology, 85: 321–5.

Royal College of Midwives (1998) Domestic abuse in pregnancy. Position Paper no. 19. RCM, London.

Scottish Office (1998) Main Findings from the 1996 Scottish Crime Survey. Stationery Office, Edinburgh.

Simpson-Subotnik L (1983) Over controlled and under controlled types of men who batter women. Paper presented at the North American meeting of the Society for Research on Aggression, Victoria, BC.

Stanko E (1997) Models of understanding violence against women. In Bewley S, Mezey G, Friend J (eds) Violence Against Women. RCOG Press, London, pp. 13–26.

Tayside Women and Violence Working Group (1994) Hit or Miss; An Exploratory Study of the Provision for Women Subjected to Domestic Violence in Tayside Region. Tayside Equal Opportunities Commission, Tayside Regional Council.

Tucker A (1995) The role of midwives in preventing domestic violence. Unpublished research project. North London College of Health Studies (now Middlesex University, School of Health, Biological and Environmental Sciences), London.

Victim Support (1992) Domestic Violence: Report of an National Interagency Working Party. London Victim Support, London.

United Kingdom Central Council for Nursing, Midwifery and Health Visiting (1992) The Scope of Professional Practice. UKCC, London.

United Kingdom Central Council for Nursing, Midwifery and Health Visiting (1996) Guidelines for Professional Practice. UKCC, London.

Yearnshire S (1997) Analysis of cohort. In Bewley S, Friend J, Mezey G (eds) Violence Against Women. RCOG Press, London, pp. 45–52.
Young A, McFarlane J (1991) Preventing abuse during pregnancy: a national educational model for health providers. Journal of Nurse Education 30: 202–6.

■ Suggested further reading

Kingston P, Penhale B (1995) Family Violence and the Caring Professions. Macmillan, Basingstoke.
Royal College of Midwives (1998) Domestic Abuse in Pregnancy Position Paper, no. 19. RCM, London.

Chapter 8

Empowerment – a gift bestowed or withheld?

Gillian Fletcher and Elisabeth Buggins

■ Introduction

Pregnancy, birth and parenthood represent a unique and powerful journey for a woman, a journey that affects her for ever. She experiences many physical, social and emotional challenges as her relationship with her partner and her status within her family and social context change. The Winterton report (House of Commons Health Committee 1992) challenged the pattern of maternity service provision based on a medical model of care. The report stated:

> that becoming a mother is not an illness... it is the mother who gives birth and who will have the lifelong commitment which motherhood brings. She is the most active participant in the birth process. (v)

In order to be an active participant, the woman needs to enter into an active partnership with the health professionals who care for her. The midwife is therefore in an ideal position to work with women throughout their journey towards motherhood, encouraging them to trust their instincts and abilities, enabling them to feel empowered and confident. Achieving empowerment in practice is not easy and may require a major reappraisal of the midwife's style of working, her perceptions of her own power and her relationship with the women in her care.

In order to empower others, one needs to feel self-confident and empowered oneself. This chapter suggests ways for the midwife to reflect on her own practice, both privately and in discussion with colleagues, to explore her own degree of empowerment and to identify the ways in which she empowers the women for whom she cares.

Kate Jackson, writing about the history of the *Changing Childbirth* strategy, suggested that:

some people perceived it to be a charter for the midwife – designed to empower her to reclaim her role as an independent and autonomous practitioner.

(Jackson 1996: 3)

Many midwives might question whether it has been an empowering experience as they struggle to implement the changes suggested by *Changing Childbirth* (DoH 1993) in a climate of resistance to change, inevitable financial constraints and, possibly, little managerial support (Gillen 1995; Henderson 1995; Sandall 1995). Sandall's study of the impact of *Changing Childbirth* on midwives identified a lack of control over how they worked rather than the workload *per se* being strongly linked to the stress they experienced (Sandall 1996).

This chapter explores the concept of empowerment in relation to a number of different issues such as:

● The medicalisation of the birth process;

● Issues of control (choices and decision-making);

● Midwifery care – art or science?

● Language and communication;

● User involvement as a means of improving services;

● Midwifery supervision.

To enable readers to reflect on the way in which their own midwifery practice mirrors or contrasts with the section they have just read, the practice checklist appears in each section rather than at the end of the chapter.

■ It is assumed that you are already aware of the following:

● The normal physiological and psychological processes of pregnancy, labour and the postnatal period;

● The basic differences between a maternity service that is based on the medical model of care and a women-centred midwifery service;

● The principles of *Changing Childbirth* (DoH 1993);

● The existence and general purpose of Maternity Services Liaison Committees (MSLCs) (see NHSE 1996).

■ What is empowerment?

Empowerment is a concept much talked about in the literature surrounding childbirth as well as in other fields, such as health promotion and social work (Ewles & Simnett 1993; Braye & Preston-Shoot 1995). The differing perspectives and definitions used in other disciplines may be helpful to midwives in broadening their understanding.

The *Oxford English Dictionary* defines the verb to empower as 'to authorise or enable a person to do'. This definition suggests a relationship in which there is an imbalance of power – one in which an individual has the ability to give or allow another to do something. In contrast, many of the working definitions in the literature on empowerment suggest more of a process in which an individual acquires or assumes power, emphasising the ability of individuals to take control of their own lives. Empowerment happens not just because powerful people give away power but because oppressed people engage in wresting it away from them, speaking out against abuse and for change (Braye & Preston-Shoot 1995: 100).

Thus, the concept of empowerment inevitably raises questions about the nature of power and power relationships, and consequently issues of ownership. Relationships are influenced by each individual's perceptions of who holds power – whether the power possessed by one is *conferred* upon the other and therefore can be given away or withheld, or is *imposed* upon the other and therefore needs to be resisted or submitted to.

In our society, health professionals are perceived as having authority (professional power): the power to save lives as well as the status to which their lengthy training, superior knowledge and expertise entitle them. Challenging the 'doctor knows best' culture is not easy for many people, yet in order to achieve true partnership, it is vital that women are equal partners in decision-making. The pregnant woman needs to be able to question treatment being offered to her if she feels that her needs and feelings are not being taken into consideration or if the care being proposed is not based on up-to-date evidence. For example, a woman is told that because her baby is lying in a breech position, she *must* have a caesarean section. She has read that, unless there are specific contraindications, the evidence suggests that she should be offered external cephalic version at 37 weeks (MIDIRS 1997). For this woman, the challenge is in trying to resolve these conflicting messages.

The relationship is made even more difficult if a woman's questions are met with resistance and a defensive response from a health professional who may be feeling insecure and threatened by this 'different approach'. One example outlined below (related to one of the authors at an antenatal class) illustrates this:

Doctor (having examined the woman who is 39 weeks pregnant) 'You will need to come in tomorrow to be induced.'
Woman 'Why do you want to induce me?'
Doctor (somewhat aggressively) 'Why don't you want to be induced?'

This woman's simple request for information was misinterpreted as a refusal of the doctor's suggested treament and a challenge to his expertise. His defensive response was clearly designed to show her who was in control. Fortunately, the woman concerned was assertive enough to state that she was not refusing to be induced but merely asking for more information about why it was necessary so that she could be involved in any decisions. Many other women would have been intimidated by the aggressive response. An individual woman will only be truly empowered when she has a real say in decisions that affect her and her baby and when communication with health professionals is based on mutual respect:

> Empowerment is not something given but something which emanates from the self. It is not an entity distributed through a chain of command but a willingness and a drive to act professionally and responsibly, grounded in a sense of self-esteem, competence and autonomy.
>
> (Osterman & Kottkamp 1993: 186)

This definition places the individual at the centre of the concept of empowerment. It implies that empowerment relies as much on self-esteem and confidence in one's own knowledge, instincts and abilities as in another person's behaving in a way that enables one to feel empowered. It might be argued that both these aspects are necessary in a relationship where the perceived balance of power, knowledge and expertise is such an unequal one, as occurs in the traditional doctor–patient relationship.

Pregnancy and birth may prove to be a time when a woman can assert control over her life and, as a result, find it a challenging and empowering experience. In order to achieve this, she will certainly need health professionals who understand the concept of empowerment and who aim to remove some of the many barriers to its achievement. To feel empowered a pregnant or labouring women needs:

- Clear unbiased information, communicated in an accessible form;
- To be trusted to make her own decisions and choices;
- To be treated with respect;
- To be listened to;
- To experience non-judgemental attitudes;
- To be encouraged and motivated;
- An empowering, enabling attitude from professionals.

What we have chosen to call an 'expert advisor model' of care encourages passivity and dependency, relying on the professional to define individual or group needs, offering solutions for them and giving advice;

while a 'partner model' encourages autonomy and empowerment by encouraging individuals to identify their own needs and exploring the possible options with them by actively listening to what is important for them (Ewles & Simnett 1993). Experts identifying and defining the needs of people in their care may neither identify nor give the same priority to the needs that those people might define as important for themselves.

Proctor (1998) compared the perceptions of women and midwives of what constitutes quality in the maternity services. The findings suggest some key differences, including midwives 'underestimating the importance of information antenatally and postnatally, the importance of continuity during labour, need for control and confidence in adjusting to the maternal role, and involvement of the woman's partner in delivery of care' (Proctor 1998: 85).

■ Practice check

● How do you know what a woman likes or needs?

● Do you offer a woman your solutions to her difficulties or explore options together?

● Whose responsibility is it to make final decisions? Do you consider that decision-making is a partnership?

● Where does the boundary lie between professional and organisational accountability and complying with the wishes of individual women?

● What do you do specifically to empower the women for whom you care?

■ Medicalisation of the birth process: professionals' attitudes and the hospital environment

The medical model of pregnancy and childbirth has for so long been the dominant one that many people today may well be forgiven for questioning the statement that 'Birth is not an illness', a principle enshrined in both the World Health Organisation report (WHO 1985) and the Winterton report (House of Commons Health Committee 1992).

The crisis, drama and heroic rescuing by clever and skilful doctors that surrounds so many television births, for example, reinforces the perception of birth as a medical event; in doing so, it undermines the central role of the midwife as the expert practitioner and undervalues the very nature of the birth process itself (Clement 1997).

Much has been written about the medicalisation of pregnancy and birth and the impact that it has had in removing women's autonomy and control over the birth process (Odent 1984; Kitzinger 1988; Raphael-Leff 1991;

Oakley 1993; Wagner 1994). Midwives too have been disempowered by this process. Many, working in high-tech environments, have lost sight of what truly constitutes 'normal labour', surrounded as they are by the ethos of pathology: that all labouring women are 'at risk' and that labour is only normal in retrospect. This preoccupation with risk has other implications. Oakley (1993) suggests that if one treats women as high risk, they are inclined to become so, while Enkin *et al* (1995) observe that fear, pain and anxiety may be increased by the mechanised clinical environment and unknown attendants, with potentially adverse effects on labour.

A woman whose first two children are now young adults highlights the impact that health professionals' attitudes can have:

> In previous pregnancies I felt 'done to' – having little explained, no choices and treated with little or no respect. My age and *naïveté* prevented me from asking questions and I therefore accepted my lot. Now I feel as if my child has been mine from conception. I've been encouraged quite rightly to take responsibility and make decisions from the start and I have felt respected. I feel this is a good start to enabling parents to take responsibility for their children.
>
> (Garcia *et al* 1998: 75)

This account highlights the importance for a woman's experience of birth of being able to take responsibility and make decisions for herself – capacities usually denied to women by medicalised maternity care. The interconnections between women's confidence and their sense of control are addressed by Goer (1996) and Gibson (1995).

Goer (1996) recognises the importance of building self-confidence by treating women as capable and competent to choose whatever they believe is best for themselves. This not only empowers them to make informed decisions, but also helps them to assume responsibility for their health and to trust their inner wisdom. This is also reflected in Gibson's (1995) definition of empowerment, which states that it is a social process of recognising, promoting and enhancing people's abilities to meet their own needs, solve their own problems and mobilise the necessary resources in order to feel in control of their lives.

■ Practice check

Imagine a group of women and their partners on a tour to familiarise them with the delivery room and postnatal wards.

- Does the experience encourage them to think in terms of partnership and autonomy or does it reinforce a medical model of childbirth, encouraging them to step fully into 'patient mode', thereby handing themselves over into the expert care of professionals to be 'rescued'?

- Does the language used encourage partnership and enable people:
  - To choose various labour positions and have a say in how the room is arranged?
  - To be fully informed partners in any decisions about pain relief and interventions?
  - To ask for the information and support they need during and after the birth?

In attempting to empower women, midwives face the challenge of overcoming cultural conditioning about birth. They have to balance a woman's possible need for reassurance with any actions or words that they might inadvertently use that will reinforce the pathological, passive, medical model of birth.

■ Issues of control

In a prospective study of 825 women booked for delivery in six hospitals in south-east England, Green *et al* (1998) explored the issue of control as it impacts on women's birth experiences.

The women in the study were sent three questionnaires: two antenatally and one postnatally.The questionnaires covered aspects such as hopes and expectations for labour, pain relief and issues of control. The response rate was 92 per cent antenatally and 96 per cent postnatally. The psychological outcome measures used were fulfilment, satisfaction with birth, emotional well-being and a description of the baby (using a 16-adjective checklist).

This study explored the concepts of choice and control, both external and internal. *External control* was defined as having control over decision-making and staff activity. It was measured by asking women for their views on having an active part in non-emergency and emergency decisions as well as how much control they expected to have and felt they had had over what staff might do or did to them. *Internal control* was defined as self-control and was explored by asking women about the control of their own behaviour, control during contractions and not making a lot of noise. The study, using a scoring system for several questions, also attempted to identify how much control women would like. Women were categorised as being 'low control' if they expressed no desire to be in control and 'high control' if they consistently expressed a strong desire to be in control. The distribution of multiparous and nulliparous women within the low control group was virtually identical to that of the whole sample (62 per cent versus 38 per cent). In the high control group, there was a higher proportion of nulliparous women (47 per cent), but the difference was not statistically significant.

The results reflect the importance for women of information and feeling in control, not only for the experience of labour, but also for their subsequent well-being. Those women who felt that they had been given the right amount of information throughout, who felt that nothing was confusing or incomplete, scored significantly better on all four psychological outcome measures. Women who did not feel in control, either of themselves or of their environment, were the least satisfied and the least likely to feel fulfilled, displaying low postnatal emotional well-being. Green *et al* (1998) comment that some women who experienced major interventions were still able to feel in control, and it is interesting to reflect on what the carers might have been doing to maintain the women's self-confidence and feelings of control even in a difficult labour.

Green *et al* (1998) acknowledge the difficulties faced in measuring satisfaction, and the chosen methodology went some way towards addressing these difficulties. The findings indicate that many common stereotypes did not hold true. Less-educated women did not want to hand over control to the staff, and the level of education did not influence how likely a woman was to subscribe to the ideal of avoiding drugs in labour. Perhaps a surprising finding was that women with low expectations were more likely to have poor psychological outcomes.

■ Midwifery care – art or science?

Enkin described the art of childbirth as those essential but unmeasurable components of care that count even though they cannot be counted, the empathy and judgement that permit care to be personalised for each woman and her family (Enkin 1989).

A small study in Iceland (Halldörsdöttir & Karlsdöttir 1996) used a phenomenonological perspective to explore the essential structure of caring or uncaring/empowering or discouraging (disempowering) birth encounters. Because of the small number of women in the study (10) and the cultural and social differences, it is not possible to generalise from the findings. However, the study raises some interesting points for further reflection on the qualities that make the midwife appear caring, sensitive and empowering.

The women cited several qualities in the caring midwife that enabled them to feel empowered, for example instinctively sensing what the woman needed and responding sensitively to those needs, being attentive and competent, truly listening as well as answering questions, having a genuine concern for the woman and her partner, showing solidarity and giving of herself – 'she shared our joy' (Halldörsdöttir & Karlsdöttir 1996: 367).

In contrast, the midwife perceived as uncaring and disempowering was indifferent, demonstrated a lack of respect for the woman as a person, did not take the initiative when that was needed, behaved thoughtlessly, was strict on routine and rules, and was domineering, coercive, indifferent and untouched by the experience – 'she felt she knew everything best herself' (Halldörsdöttir & Karlsdöttir 1996: 371).

The authors reflect that the need for caring encounters for women giving birth in a technological environment is paramount and suggest that midwives need to promote both the art and the science of midwifery (Halldórsdóttir & Karlsdóttir 1996).

Similar key themes, such as respecting the mother's wishes, the midwife sharing her own experience, being a good listener, friendly, approachable, non-critical and non-judgemental, also emerged from a study that asked 115 women what made a good midwife (Pope *et al* 1998).

The concept of power is explored by Bianchi (1995). She highlights the difficulty that the woman in labour faces in trying to maintain her authority and influence over the situation in a strange and medicalised environment where what happens is strongly influenced by the authority that the health professionals have over her. They can easily persuade the woman to do things that would not have been her chosen course of action. An example of this is a woman keen to remain mobile in labour who gets on to the bed to be monitored on arrival in hospital and becomes immobilised.

■ Practice check

Read the paragraphs below and reflect on the way in which the highlighted phrases and terminology may reinforce feelings of passivity in a woman.

> On *admission* to hospital in labour, a woman is told that the midwife will *check* her over. When she arrives, she is asked to *'pop up on the bed'*, where the midwife will *put her* on a monitor to check the baby, and *if everything is all right*, she will *be allowed* to get up and walk around. When she is examined, the women might be told, 'Oh dear I'm afraid you're *only* 3 cm dilated. A long way to go yet.'

> She will *be allowed* to have a bath if her waters have not broken or there is no meconium staining. She is told that *when things get too painful,* she can have pethidine or an epidural as long as she does not leave it too late. Later, she might be told that because of *failure to progress or because the baby is distressed,* she *needs* the doctor to *deliver the baby.* He will tell them whether or not her partner will *be allowed* to stay if an assisted delivery is necessary.

> On the postnatal ward, she *tries* to breastfeed and possibly has someone who *helps* her latch the baby on, that is, *puts her baby on the breast for her*. She gets somewhat tearful when it is suggested that because her baby is *crying a lot*, she has to give him a bottle. She will *be discharged or allowed to go home* on day two.

Work with colleagues and rewrite the above scenario, substituting empowering words that can boost a woman's confidence in her ability to give birth and parent effectively.

■ Language – empowering or disempowering

The language of pregnancy and birth is something that is easily taken for granted. It is likely to be so familiar and so much a part of a midwife's day-to-day work that it is useful to reflect on what images certain words might be conveying to the pregnant woman and her partner at a subconscious, if not conscious, level. Many of the phrases and terms used (for example, '*incompetent* cervix', '*failure to progress*', and '*trial* of labour') can so easily create an image of helplessness and inadequacy of the female body to achieve the momentous task of birth (Smith 1993; Buggins 1995). Language can inadvertently reinforce the woman's fears and anxieties about the dangers of birth and do little to instil confidence in the wonderfully powerful ability of the female body to nurture and give birth to a baby.

Although an examination may be routine to the midwife, it is likely to have great significance for the woman and her family. Following an antenatal visit, the woman is likely to be asked what was said to her at the clinic, and she needs to be able to reassure her family that all is well (Flint 1994). Women interpret the words of midwives and doctors in ways that may not be realised.

'You're growing well, the baby's nice and big...' may result in the fear that it will never get out. Alternatively, a midwife who tells a pregnant woman that if she continues to smoke during her pregnancy her baby will be born small for dates might be surprised to discover that this was perceived by the women as being beneficial in that it is easier to give birth to a *small* baby. As with the previous checklist, you might like to reflect on the words that you and your colleagues regularly use when working with pregnant women.

■ User involvement in maternity service planning and monitoring

User involvement in the development of services, together with a multi-disciplinary approach to service planning is essential if maternity services are to reflect the needs and views of those who use them.

(Winyard & Moores 1996)

There are many different ways in which midwives can find out what women need from maternity services. Different approaches such as parent panels and Maternity Services Liaison Committee (MSLC)-initiated user groups have been discussed by Gready *et al* (1997).

Service user involvement in the committees set up to develop and monitor maternity services since 1984 (Maternity Care in Action 1984) has been an important development. In the early days, there was often only one lone woman serving as a user representative on the MSLC, and the committees were often only exchanging information about decisions made elsewhere rather than being actively involved in service planning (personal communication from VOICES trainees; this project is described below.)

In 1996, new guidelines (NHSE 1996) strengthened and clarified the position of MSLCs as independent advisory bodies that have a key role in successful implementation of the *Changing Childbirth* programme. The guidelines recommended that, in every health authority, there needs to be an effective MSLC, with a lay chair, in which commissioners, providers and users work in partnership to develop services.

The NCT VOICES project (Fletcher *et al* 1997), funded by the Department of Health, investigated how MSLC and Community Health Council user representatives could be facilitated to carry out their role more effectively and developed a training programme to meet the needs identified. Questionnaires were sent to 379 existing user representatives; 169 returns (45 per cent) were analysed. The representatives were asked a number of questions relating to their work on MSLCs, for example on the level of participation and work with others on the committee, including questions about how knowledgeable and confident they felt in their role. Over two-thirds of the respondents felt confident about putting an item on the agenda (68 per cent) and asking a question in the meetings (74 per cent), whereas only half felt confident about presenting evidence (47 per cent) or keeping the attention focused on issues of importance (50 per cent). When asked about the challenges they faced, the greatest number volunteered that it was feeling accepted and being taken seriously. How to bring about change and to represent other parents' views were identified as being the most important training needs (Fletcher *et al* 1997).

The VOICES training included many activities that explored relationships and communication between health professionals and users, and aimed to develop skills empowering and enabling women to represent the views of their peers and to effectively make a case for change.

A number of the women attending the VOICES training were chairpersons of their local MSLCs, in accordance with the NHSE guidelines. One might think that women willing to take on such a challenging and important role feel empowered and confident. However, many expressed frustration at the difficulties they faced:

> 'I find that chairing this multidisciplinary committee is one of the most challenging and difficult tasks I have undertaken in a long time. It is hard to be one of only two other user representatives when all the other members of the committee are people who know each other and work together, often on a daily basis. But when you hear local mothers praising something about the maternity services in which you played a part it all seems very worthwhile.'
>
> (Buggins *et al* 1996: 541)

One woman talked of having been a member of the committee for 7 years and yet some of the medical staff still did not address her by name:

'The minutes of the meetings constantly quote medical/management staff by their name. Any points that I or other lay members make are referred to in the minutes as "It was pointed out that..."'.

(Buggins *et al* 1996: 541)

The results of the study highlight the unequal power base that service users continue to face and the subtle ways in which health professionals can disempower them. When asked how the training had influenced the way in which they related to other committee members, the most frequently cited changes were:

- Seeing professionals now as equals;

- Having the confidence to speak out;

- An increased awareness of the difficulties that professionals face;

- Relating better to other users.

Women who have been through the training feel more confident and assertive. This shifts the balance of power in the relationship between health professionals and service users, mentioned earlier in this chapter, and health professionals may find themselves feeling threatened. New ways of working together will have to be found.

Recruiting users to MSLCs and regularly seeking out the views of service users is not easy. Women with disabilites, young mothers and those from ethnic minority groups are currently underrepresented on these committees. If the services are to be truly women centred, it is important that users themselves play a part in the planning and monitoring process.

■ Practice check

- Are you a midwife member of an MSLC? If not a member yourself, do you receive feedback from the local midwife representative?

- What aspects of care are discussed at your local MSLC meetings?

- Do you see a copy of the minutes of the meetings?

- Are you able to suggest items for the agenda?

- How many user members does your local MSLC have? Perhaps it has a separate user subgroup that regularly meets with groups of midwives to discuss aspects of care. Could you attend a meeting?

- How do you work in partnership with users to develop services that are truly women centred?

■ Supervision

Cathy Warwick observes that 'Normally... high standards will emerge more effectively if midwives are treated themselves as they are expected to treat women' (Warwick 1996: 112). The philosophy informing the supervision of midwifery practice at Kings College Hospital, London, that she outlines, links very clearly with some of the issues explored in this chapter. Warwick suggests that supervision should be conducted in a way that enables midwives to grow and develop. Good supervision requires a climate encouraging openness and honesty, and engendering a sense of trust and an ability to acknowledge and explore strengths, weaknesses and prejudices. Only by openly exploring prejudices can attitudes change and a more woman-centred approach emerge. As part of this growing self-awareness, reflective practice and innovative ideas need to be encouraged, and hierarchical systems should be used with the objective of support rather than control.

☐ Self-reflection for supervisors

Complete the following phrases personally or with a group of colleagues:

● In order to empower the midwives whom I supervise, I need to...

● In order to feel more empowered myself, I need to...

● The barriers to empowerment are...

How often do you ask for feedback from those with whom you work about whether or not your style of working is empowering?

■ Summary

Empowerment may be said to be about letting go so that others may grow. Entering into a more equal partnership whereby women are empowered should not in any way undermine the expertise of the midwife: letting go of some of the power and sharing control does not necessarily mean losing it. The challenge for health professionals is in moving from the role of expert advisor, which may be the more familiar and comfortable one, to that of a more equal partner with specialist skills and knowledge that can be shared with women. The rewards are likely to be better communication and an improved relationship with the woman and her partner as well as less opportunity for misunderstandings and consequent litigation. Women need the knowledge and opportunity to help them to develop confidence in their own abilities and decision-making skills. In the words of Schott (1994: 4): 'Let's not leave any woman holding her baby without having conveyed to her our complete respect and belief in her ability to think clearly, make decisions and to be a good parent.'

In order to meet the challenges of working in this way, the midwife needs to feel empowered herself. As already identified earlier in this chapter, self-esteem, confidence, autonomy, affirmation, praise, encouragement, respect and having one's contributions valued are all key factors in empowerment. Confidence comes through feeling secure in one's knowledge and being able to rise to the challenge.

■ Recommendations for clinical practice in the light of currently available evidence

1. Midwives need to review their style of working with women and colleagues to ensure that they are providing the best possible opportunity to enable women to feel empowered and in control.

2. Midwives should be aware of the effects of media images on women's perceptions of chidlbirth and ensure that the language and procedures used do not reinforce the passive medical image.

3. Midwives and other professionals involved in conducting research should bear in mind that medically defined clinical outcomes may not be the only or the most important ones for women and their partners. Midwives could be more proactive in trying to ensure that the views of local women are regularly sought on what is important to women and promoting research in these areas.

4. Midwives should work closely in partnership with user and other MSLC members to ensure that women-centred services are developed.

■ References

Bianchi A (1995) Powerful or powerless: is it a mother's choice? International Journal of Childbirth Education, 11(3): 37–8.

Braye S, Preston-Shoot M (1995) Power, partnership and empowerment. In Braye S, Preston-Shoot M (eds) Empowering Practice in Social Care. Open University Press, Buckingham, pp. 98–122.

Buggins E (1995) Mind your language. Nursing Standard, 10(1): 22.

Buggins E, Newburn M, Fletcher G, Gready M, Draper J, Dodds R (1996) Finding our voices. British Journal of Midwifery, 4(10): 539–42.

Clement S (1997) Childbirth on television. British Journal of Midwifery, 5(1): 37–42.

Department of Health (1993) Changing Childbirth Part I. Report of the Expert Maternity Group. HMSO, London.

Enkin M (1989) Effective care of the low risk woman in pregnancy and childbirth. Women's Health in the 1990s. Conference proceedings of 9th International Congress of Psychosomatic Obstetrics and Gynaecology, Amsterdam, May 1989. Parthenon, Lancashire.

Enkin M, Keirse M, Chalmers I (1995) A Guide to Effective Care in Pregnancy and Childbirth. Oxford University Press, Oxford.

Ewles L, Simnett I (1993) Fundamentals of communication. In Promoting Health – a Practical Guide, 2nd edn. Scutari Press, London, pp. 121–38.

Fletcher G, Buggins E, Newburn M, Gready M, Draper J, Wang M (1997) The Voices Project Final Report. National Childbirth Trust, London.

Garcia J, Redshaw M, Fitzsimons B, Keene J (1998) First Class Delivery. A National Survey of Women's Views of Maternity Care. Audit Commission, London.

Gibson CH (1995) Definitions of empowerment. Handout 1.7. In RCM Invest in Breast Together. RCM, London.

Gillen J (1995) Can midwives practice autonomously? British Journal of Midwifery, 3(5): 245–6.

Goer H (1996) Childbirth education empowers women to make informed choices in health care, to assume responsibility for their health and to trust their inner wisdom. Journal of Perinatal Education, 1: 11–12.

Gready M, Buggins E, Newburn M, Fletcher G, Dodds R, Wang M (1997) Hearing it like it is: understanding the views of users. British Journal of Midwifery, 5(8): 496–500.

Green J, Coupland V, Kitzinger J (1998) Great Expectations. A Prospective Study of Women's Expectations and Experiences of Childbirth. Books for Midwives Press, Hale.

Halldórsdóttir S, Karlsdóttir S (1996) Empowerment or discouragement: women's experiences of caring and uncaring encounters during childbirth. Health Care for Women International, 17: 361–79.

Henderson C (1995) All change. British Journal of Midwifery, 3(12): 630–1.

House of Commons Health Committee (1992) Second Report, Maternity Services vol. 1, Section 100. HMSO, London.

Jackson K (1996) History of changing childbirth. In Dodds R, Goodman M, Tyler S (eds) Listen with Mother. Books for Midwives Press, Hale, p. 3.

Kitzinger S (1988) Why women need midwives. In Kitzinger S (ed.) The Midwife Challenge. Pandora, London, pp. 1–20.

Maternity Care in Action (1984) Part 2. HMSO, London.

MIDIRS (1997) Breech Presentation – Options for Care. Informed Choice for Women. MIDIRS/NHS Centre for Reviews and Dissemination, Bristol.

NHSE (1996) Maternity Services Liaison Committees – Guidelines for Working Effectively. DoH, London.

Oakley A (1993) Birth as a Normal Process. Essays on Women, Medicine and Health. Edinburgh University Press, Edinburgh.

Odent M (1984) Birth Reborn. What Childbirth Should Be. Souvenir Press, London.

Osterman KF and Kottkamp RB (1993) Reflective practice for educators. Cited in Furneaux N (1995) Achieving professional empowerment through education. The challenge of changing childbirth. Midwifery Educational Resource Pack. ENB, London.

Pope R, Cooney M, Graham L, Holliday M, Patel S (1998) Aspects of care: 4. Views of professionals and mothers. British Journal of Midwifery, 6 (3): 144–7.

Proctor S (1998) What determines quality in maternity care? Comparing perceptions of childbearing women and midwives. Birth, 25: 85.

Raphael-Leff J (1991) Psychological Processes of Childbearing. Chapman & Hall, London.

Sandall J (1995) Burnout and midwifery: an occupational hazard? British Journal of Midwifery 3(5): 620–1.

Sandall J (1996) Moving towards caseload practice: what evidence do we have? British Journal of Midwifery, 4(12): 246–8.

Schott J (1994) The importance of encouraging women to think for themselves. British Journal of Midwifery, 2(1): 3–4.

Smith A (1993) The meaning behind the WORDS. New Generation, 12(2): 15.

Wagner M (1994) Pursuing the Birth Machine. ACE Graphics, Camperdown, Australia.

Warwick C (1996) Supervision and practice change at King's. In Kirkham M (ed.) Supervision of Midwives. Books for Midwives Press, Hale.

WHO (1985) Birth is not an illness. 15 Recommendations of the World Heath Organisation. WHO Report on Appropriate Technology for Birth. WHO, Geneva.

Winyard G, Moores Y (1996) Covering Letter: Maternity Services Liaison Committees – Guidelines for Working Effectively. NHSE, Leeds.

■ Suggested further reading

Craig G. (1998) Women's Views Count – Building responsive maternity services. A resource pack to help health professionals and user representatives ask service users their views. College of Health. London.

Green J, Coupland V, Kitzinger J (1998) Great Expectations. A Prospective Study of Women's Expectations and Experiences of Childbirth. Books for Midwives Press. Hale.

Robertson A (1997) Empowering women. Teaching Active Birth in the 90s. ACE Graphics, Camperdown, Australia.

Chapter 9

Organisation of postnatal care and related issues

Debra Bick

■ Introduction

> It is clear to us from the evidence of the professions that postnatal care, like other aspects of the maternity services, is poorly evaluated and researched, delivered in often inappropriate and fragmented ways and has a dissipated managerial focus which militates against efficient use of resources.
>
> (House of Commons Health Committee 1992: xcvi)

This chapter examines the organisation of hospital- and community-based care during the postnatal period. Studies that have examined the organisation of postnatal services across the UK are discussed, and the need for evidence of the benefit and effectiveness of the current organisation of care is emphasised throughout the chapter. Related issues include the historical background of midwifery postnatal care, the duration of postnatal visits, the content of care, the role of other members of the primary health care team during the postnatal period and maternal morbidity. Studies of alternative models of postnatal organisation currently in progress are referred to at the end of the chapter.

■ It is assumed that you are already aware of the following:

- The current pattern of postnatal home visits that a woman will receive from her midwife, health visitor and GP;

- The statutory responsibility of the midwife during the postnatal period;

- The routine content of postnatal midwifery care;

- Common health problems experienced by women following childbirth;

- The aim of the final consultation that a woman is offered with her GP 6–8 weeks postnatally.

■ Historical background to the organisation of postnatal care

The pattern and content of postnatal care were established over 80 years ago when maternal mortality, as a result of complications following childbirth, was high. At the beginning of the 20th century, the maternal death rate was 4 per 1000 births, the majority of women dying from puerperal infection (Towler & Bramall 1986). Postnatal care was therefore focused on the prevention of infection, and this demanded a high level of 'nursing' care from the midwife (Abbott *et al* 1997).

Up to the late 1940s, the majority of births in the UK took place at home, following which a period of 'lying in' occurred when the woman was 'confined' to bed to recuperate following the birth. The duration of the 'lying in' period often depended on a woman's circumstances, but the first Midwives Act of 1902, which formalised the organisation and regulation of midwives through the instigation of the Central Midwives Board, established 10 days as the minimum number of days that a woman should 'lie in'. For these 10 days, the woman was expected to rest and receive attention from a midwife (Ball 1994), who was expected, among her other duties, to bathe both mother and baby on a daily basis (Leap & Hunter 1993).

The gradual medicalisation of childbirth and the move for all women to give birth in hospital on the grounds of 'safety' (Campbell & Macfarlane 1994) focused the role of the community midwife on postnatal care. However, despite a continued adherence to a rigid policy of postnatal home visits, limited information was available on the role of midwives during the postnatal period. As Campbell and Macfarlane (1994) noted, after 1987 the only data collected nationally on the work of community midwives concerned the number of 'face-to-face' contacts that they made, with no mention of the purpose of visits. Prior to this, the data collected specified whether visits had been made to antenatal or postnatal women.

The transfer of place of delivery from home to hospital led to postnatal care becoming more organised around 'time targets'. In addition to the minimum number of days that a woman should be visited by a midwife, time targets established the minimum number of days that a woman should remain on the hospital postnatal ward, when she should receive a first home visit from her health visitor and when she should be seen for a final consultation with her GP and discharged from the maternity services. As Ball (1994) highlighted, there was no basis on which to assume that any period could be considered as the 'proper' time within which a woman should have adapted to being a new mother. Yet postnatal care continues to be organised on the assumption that a woman has recovered, and can cope with all the extra demands that parenthood places upon her, within 6–8 weeks of giving birth.

■ The organisation of hospital postnatal care

For the majority of women, postnatal care commences on the delivery suite, where they will remain after giving birth for a variable length of time until transferred to the postnatal ward. Care on the postnatal ward is usually organised around activities such as doctors' ward rounds, midwives' shift patterns and the number of midwives and support staff (auxiliary nurses and nursery nurses) on duty. The organisation and layout of postnatal wards varies between maternity hospitals. Women admitted to designated postnatal wards may have an experience of care different from those admitted to wards that take antenatal and postnatal women, where midwives may have to give priority to women admitted with antenatal complications or in early labour.

Each hospital will have policies regarding the length of time that a woman is 'allowed' to stay that are generally based on the type of delivery a woman has had and the time of day during a 24-hour period that she gave birth (Ball 1994). The average length of hospital postnatal stay has gradually decreased. In 1981, the average postnatal stay for all deliveries was 5.4 days, although this figure varied from region to region (Rider 1984). In 1997, the average length of stay for women who had a normal delivery was 2.5 days, but this figure continues to vary between regions (Audit Commission 1997). Some variation results from the differing rates of obstetric intervention during labour (for example, the number of instrumental deliveries or emergency caesarean sections), but some is caused by the different administrative procedures in place, which include the policies that a unit has for baby checks and the protocols of individual consultant obstetricians.

Early transfer home was seen as a recognition of a shift in emphasis in the aims of postnatal care, from physical care of the woman to the provision of education, counselling and support for the woman and her family (Rider 1984). Some potential problems that could arise as a consequence of early transfer were highlighted, including difficulty in ensuring that there was adequate domestic support for the woman, the need to provide an emergency 24-hour advisory service and the diversion of monies away from hospital-based care to the community (Rider 1984). The impact of the alteration of the service on maternal well-being or the workload of community midwives does not appear to have been considered.

■ The effect of hospital postnatal stay on maternal outcomes

In a survey of the maternity services in England and Wales carried out by the Audit Commission (1997), the majority of women felt that their stay in hospital was 'about right', but 25 per cent of the 2375 women questioned reported that they were dissatisfied with this. Dissatisfaction was reported from both women who had longer lengths of stay than average and women who reported that they were discharged home before they felt ready. The Audit Commission (1997) included in their recommendations for postnatal care that the length of hospital stay should be flexible and that women should be consulted on how long they wanted to stay.

Little is known about outcomes of maternal well-being and satisfaction with care in relation to different lengths of postnatal hospital stay. A descriptive study carried out in six districts in the Yorkshire region focused on the implications of a variation in the length of stay on women's experience of care, satisfaction with care and psychological well-being (Dowswell *et al* 1997). The survey was carried out following government reports that encouraged maternity service providers to offer women more choice about their care (DoH 1993), but at a time of pressure on maternity units to reduce or keep down service costs.

One hundred and twenty randomly selected women in each health district (*n* = 720) who delivered during a specified 4-week period were asked to complete a postal questionnaire when they were 4–8 weeks postpartum. Questions were included on satisfaction with and experience of hospital postnatal care. Psychological well-being was assessed using standard measures including the Edinburgh Postnatal Depression Scale (Cox *et al* 1987). Although length of postnatal hospital stay varied significantly between the districts for women who had a normal vaginal delivery, there was no difference in women's depression scores in each district or in whether women were satisfied with their length of stay. The researchers then compared whether women themselves perceived their length of stay as appropriate, with their psychological outcome. There was a significant association between women who perceived that their length of stay had been too short and a higher depression score on the Edinburgh Postnatal Depression Scale. The researchers concluded that length of postnatal hospital stay could have implications for consumer satisfaction and maternal psychological outcomes, but hospitals could be flexible and offer women a choice about the length of stay to comply with the philosophy of *Changing Childbirth* (DoH 1993) without compromising efficiency targets (Dowswell *et al* 1997).

The environment and routine pattern of hospital postnatal care has frequently been cited as a reason for the low uptake and early cessation of breastfeeding in the UK (Woolridge 1996; Foster *et al* 1997). The Audit Commission (1997) highlighted the important contribution that Trusts had to make towards promoting breastfeeding through the way in which they organised postnatal care in hospital and the community. A review of randomised controlled trials examining the effects of early versus late discharge from hospital after birth on breastfeeding duration found that early discharge might be beneficial to the continuation of breastfeeding, particularly among multiparae (Renfrew & Lang 1998). Recent attempts to alter breastfeeding practices include the WHO/UNICEF Baby Friendly Hospital Initiative (Saadeh & Akre 1996), which aims to remove hospital practices such as restrictions on the duration of breastfeeds, the giving of supplementary formula feeds to breastfed babies and the use of pacifiers, in order to improve breastfeeding rates.

The contribution of the home environment to the successful establishment of breastfeeding will depend to a large extent on the quality of the breastfeeding support provided by the woman's family, peer group and primary health care team. Further research is necessary to examine factors associated with the home environment that influence the uptake and continuation of breastfeeding, and how the organisation of postnatal midwifery care could best support these women. Sally Inch discusses these and other breastfeeding issues in Chapter 5 of this volume.

Many complaints about hospital postnatal care have focused on the ward environment, the quality of food and poor standards of hygiene (McCourt & Page 1996; Audit Commission 1997). This has led to some calls in the midwifery press to end hospital postnatal care (Walsh 1997). However, caution has been urged before Trusts move to reorganise or reduce the availability of hospital postnatal care and thus further restrict any choice that a woman may exercise about her care without the evidence to support this (Marchant *et al* 1998; Bick *et al* 1998).

The recent changes to the organisation of midwifery care, which now include team midwifery, DOMINO schemes and individual caseloads, may have reduced some of the pressure placed on hospital midwives. However, there is limited evidence of the effect that these changes have had on the effectiveness of the postnatal care that women receive in hospital. An evaluation of three midwifery group practice development projects (Allen *et al* 1997) highlighted problems with lack of communication and co-operation between hospital midwives working on postnatal wards and midwives working in the group practices. These issues need to be addressed if women are to receive optimal postnatal care.

■ The organisation of community-based postnatal care

There is a marked variation in how midwifery services are organised in the community. For example, midwives may be organised to provide care to women registered with specific general practices, or they may care for women resident within a defined geographical area. The offices they work from may be based at their local maternity unit or a community health centre. There has been no evaluation of the organisation of midwifery community services with regard to the effect on communication with members of the primary health care team, midwives' job satisfaction or whether equitable use is made of available resources to meet the needs of the local population.

The Audit Commission (1997) reported that while postnatal visits by midwives were popular with women, their purpose was largely unspecified and there was no evidence of their clinical effectiveness. Community-based postnatal care has traditionally been organised around the provision of home visits by midwives to perform routine observations and examinations. Following birth, the postnatal period in terms of midwifery input is defined in the Midwives Rules (UKCC 1993 p. 8) as 'a period of not less than ten and not more than twenty-eight days after the end of labour, during which the continued attendance of a midwife on the mother is requisite'. Prior to 1986 daily visits until the tenth postnatal day were specified in the midwife's Code of Practice (Central Midwives Board 1983), and one of the few changes made to the organisation of midwifery care was the introduction of a policy of 'selective' postnatal visiting (UKCC 1986). However, there was no evidence to support this alteration to the pattern of care and little guidance on how selective visiting should be introduced and maintained.

A questionnaire-based survey of all health districts in England in 1991 found that the extent to which selective visiting occurred in practice was variable, and it was apparent that, in many districts, the change in the frequency of visits was minor (Garcia *et al* 1994). The questionnaire was sent to the directors of midwifery services or their equivalent in all of the then 189 NHS health districts in England; replies were received from 167 districts. Almost all of the districts had a policy of selective visits to women at home before the tenth postnatal day. Only 10 districts were adhering to the traditional policy of daily visits until the tenth day. In a further 10 districts, this policy was followed but was under review, and in nine districts the practice but not the formal policy had changed. Despite the change to the pattern of visits, there was little information provided regarding how midwives might decide to select women for fewer or more frequent visits. There was considerable variation between districts in the extent to which the new policies allowed midwives to decide on a pattern of visits.

A small ethnographic study of women's and midwives' views of the pattern of postnatal visiting highlighted discrepancies between the opinions of the 'providers' and the 'users'. (Hamilton 1998). Midwives thought that selective visiting improved the postnatal care they gave, but women reported that they were not always informed that they could be involved in decisions regarding the frequency and duration of postnatal visits and did not consider that selective visiting enhanced their care.

A small pilot project was undertaken in Glasgow to find out whether planning care to meet the individual needs of postnatal women reduced the number of problems experienced by the woman and her baby, and increased continuity of care, satisfaction with care and cost savings to the NHS (Twaddle *et al* 1993). Midwives were only given a brief agenda for action to achieve this, which consisted mainly of requiring them to plan ongoing care with the woman at the first visit.

Assessments carried out after this agenda was implemented found that, even with such a minimal plan, the midwives made significantly fewer visits and there was a reduction in the number of women seeing more than three midwives. Women were mostly satisfied with their care, and the proportion of women who felt that a daily visit was necessary dropped significantly between the two time periods. This suggested that the new type of care was more popular with the women, although there was no information on whether the actual content of care was individualised.

The pattern of postnatal visits in some areas of the UK continues to adhere to a policy of daily visits until the tenth day. A recent survey of women's views of the maternity services (Garcia *et al* 1998) asked women about the pattern of visits that they had received. A random sample of women who gave birth in England and Wales in June and July 1995 (*n* = 3570) were sent a questionnaire when their baby was around 4 months old. A response rate of 2406 (67 per cent) was obtained.

Of 2297 women who answered a question about the pattern of postnatal midwifery visits they received, 29 per cent were visited every day until day 10, 32 per cent were visited every day except one, and 29 per cent were visited every other day. The regional pattern of age of the baby at the last midwifery visit also varied considerably; in the south-east of England, 55 per cent of visits stopped at 10 days or before, but this was the case for only 28 per cent of visits in the north-west. Many women received visits from more than one midwife: 16 per cent of women were visited by one midwife only, 44 per cent saw two, and 40 per cent saw three or more.

☐ **Duration of visits**

Marsh and Sargent (1991) carried out a study in the Lothian Region of Scotland to determine which factors affected the duration of midwifery home visits. Community midwives were asked to record which of 32 factors from a given list were relevant to each visit. Using this proforma, factors were recorded by 24 midwives during a 2-week period from 783 visits made to 224 mothers. Ten factors independently influenced the duration of postnatal visits. These were grouped as 'time-consuming procedures' (physical examination of the mother; performing a PKU test; physical examination of the baby), 'administration related' (liaison with the GP, health visitor or both; the total number of visits to be made in the same day; the waiting time to see the mother; previous contact between the mother and the midwife), 'feeding related' (breastfeeding problems; previous experience of breastfeeding) and 'delivery related' (delivery complications). The concentration of the midwife on physical tasks suggested that this was a reflection of the midwife's rather than the mother's perception of need.

■ **Content of care**

The content of postnatal midwifery care traditionally consists of observations and examinations, which can include taking the woman's temperature and pulse, recording her blood pressure, examining her breasts, assessing uterine involution, observing the lochia and, if appropriate, examining her perineum.

One of the aims of providing routine midwifery observations and examinations is to detect postnatal health problems, but evidence is required to show whether these are effective or indeed whether they detect health problems now known to be commonly experienced (MacArthur *et al* 1991; Glazener *et al* 1995; see also below on 'Postpartum morbidity'). One component of routine care is abdominal palpation to assess whether uterine involution is progressing normally. A deviation from the normal is purported to be associated with morbidity such as uterine infection or secondary postpartum haemorrhage (Marchant & Garcia 1995), but there is little information on whether these conditions can be detected by performing abdominal palpation. The findings of a prospective study by Alexander *et al* (1997) that included an investigation of whether midwives' assessments of postnatal uterine involution predicted vaginal loss problems found evidence to suggest that these observations do predict which women go on to develop such problems after discharge from the midwife's care. Further research into this complex area is required.

■ The role of other health professionals during the postnatal period

In addition to receiving care from a midwife during the postnatal period, the maternity services are organised to ensure that women receive a primary visit from their health visitor between 10 and 14 days after the birth as well as the provision of one or more home visits and a final consultation with their GP at 6–8 weeks. There is little anecdotal or research evidence available to assess the impact or effectiveness of the organisation of these services.

☐ The role of the health visitor

The health visitor's role is generic, combining health surveillance, health promotion and diagnostic health screening. The primary visit in many cases coincides with the midwifery discharge of the mother, although this visit is not a statutory requirement (Kroll & Dwyer 1994). The visit is generally to offer advice and can include a discussion of contraception, infant feeding and child immunisation. If the midwife is still visiting a mother after 10 days, the health visitor may delay an initial or follow-up visit, or arrange to see the mother at the baby clinic. Health visitors in many areas administer the Edinburgh Postnatal Depression Scale to screen for depression, but the effectiveness of this service has not been evaluated.

Potential problems that arise as a consequence of a woman receiving home visits from a health visitor and a midwife during the postnatal period could include duplication of care and conflicting advice, particularly on infant feeding (RCM Scotland & Scottish HVA 1995). Research into ways of enhancing collaborative practice between midwives and health visitors is urgently required.

☐ The role of the GP

A woman may receive a number of home visits from her GP, the first visit usually being made within a day or two of hospital discharge. There is no information on how many women receive GP home visits, the number of visits made or what benefits, if any, accrue to the woman or her family from such visits during this period. These are issues that need to be addressed.

A postnatal check at 6–8 weeks is offered to the majority of women. This marks the end of the puerperium and discharge from the maternity services. Uptake for this consultation is high: 88 per cent in a study in Oldham (Bowers 1985) and 91 per cent in a study in Birmingham (Bick & MacArthur 1995a). The content of this visit has recently been questioned (Sharif *et al* 1993). Sharif *et al* studied the GP records of 125 women who had routine vaginal examination as part of their 6–8-week check and found that only six women had any abnormality detected, none of these requiring treatment. Contraceptive advice is frequently offered at the postnatal discharge visit, yet recent work in Scotland (Glazener 1997) has shown that more than half of women will have resumed sexual intercourse by the sixth week. A discussion of contraception at this visit is clearly too late.

■ Postpartum morbidity

Until recently, there had been little systematic research into morbidity following childbirth, with the exception of studies of postnatal depression (Kumar & Robson 1984; Cox *et al* 1987). MacArthur *et al* in Birmingham (1991) first documented the occurrence of substantial physical postpartum morbidity, largely unreported to health professionals and persisting well beyond the 6-week routine maternity discharge. This study of over 11,000 women identified widespread morbidity starting after childbirth. As many as 47 per cent of the women reported one or more of a list of 25 health problems beginning for the first time after birth and lasting for more than 6 weeks. Over 60 per cent of the problems were still present at questioning between 1 and 9 years after giving birth, indicating that many of the symptoms became chronic. Few women reported these health problems to their GP.

Researchers in other centres confirmed this widespread and persistent morbidity. Glazener *et al* (1995), in a study of over 1200 women who comprised a 20 per cent random sample of deliveries during 1 year in Grampian, Scotland, found that 76 per cent of women experienced at least one health problem 8 weeks after delivery. A small study of postnatal care in two districts in London (Garcia & Marchant 1993) found that, at 8 weeks postpartum, 23 per cent of 90 women had headaches, 20 per cent backache and 22 per cent constipation, and 39 per cent felt low or depressed since giving birth.

A subsequent study in Birmingham that examined the severity and impact of postpartum morbidity found that, although some health problems are only slight or occur intermittently, many women suffer symptoms daily, some of which have a significant effect on various aspects of their lives (Bick & MacArthur 1995b).

■ Research in progress examining different models of the organisation of postnatal care

The current organisation of postnatal care may not be appropriate to identify and manage health problems now known to be commonly experienced by women after childbirth (MacArthur *et al* 1991; Glazener *et al* 1995), but there is little information on this. Following the recent government reports stating the need for wide-ranging changes to the maternity services (House of Commons Health Committee 1992; DoH 1993), a randomised controlled trial is in progress to compare current postnatal care with a new model of protocol-based, midwifery-led care (Bick *et al* 1997). Forty general practices throughout the West Midlands health region have been randomised so that the midwives attached to the practices will provide either current care (control) or new model care (intervention).

Women in the control arm will receive postnatal care in line with current practice. The focus of visits in the intervention arm is the identification and management of physical and psychological postnatal health problems. Midwives in this arm will plan the frequency and timing of visits with each woman at the first postnatal home contact. A symptom checklist will be used on two occasions to identify problems, since earlier studies have shown that women do not spontaneously report these (MacArthur *et al* 1991; Bick & MacArthur 1995b). Ten sets of evidence-based and peer-reviewed guidelines will be implemented by the midwife to manage identified problems appropriately. All women will receive intermittent home visits until the 28th day and a final consultation with the midwife at 10–12 weeks. This is intended to replace the GP 6–8-week check where appropriate and will also focus on the identification and management of symptoms. Deferring this consultation may provide more time for women to consider their own health needs, rather than just those of their baby.

At 4 months and 12 months after the birth, all women will receive a postal questionnaire, which will include two validated health measures (the SF36 and the Edinburgh Postnatal Depression Scale) to assess their physical and psychological well-being. Cost-effectiveness analysis will be undertaken to compare the resource use and resource requirements of the current versus the new care. It is important to determine the effect on all relevant health professionals of any reorganisation of the maternity services (Garcia *et al*

1997). Therefore, the views of midwives, health visitors and GPs from all the practices will be sought at the end of the trial. The trial will provide, for the first time, detailed information regarding the effects and benefits of the current organisation of postnatal care as well as a new model of care.

A recent randomised controlled trial in Sheffield has evaluated the effectiveness of a new model of support for women in the early postnatal period compared with the current organisation of midwifery care (Morrell *et al* 1997). This model is based on the Dutch organisation of postnatal care. In the Netherlands, midwives work with an assistant, known as a maternity aide nurse, whose role includes assisting the midwife at home deliveries and the provision of postnatal care, supervised by the midwife (Fillmore & Miedema 1996). Postnatal duties include monitoring the woman's and infant's health, assistance with the feeding and general care of the baby, and teaching parenthood skills.

Women in the Sheffield trial who were randomised to receive a community support worker were offered visits in addition to midwifery care. Visits were offered for a maximum of 3 hours a day, with a total of 10 visits during the first 28 days after delivery. The support worker's remit was to promote rest and recuperation by providing practical help and care for other children, providing companionship and support for the woman and promoting confidence in the woman's adaptation to parenthood. Outcome measures are maternal physical and psychological health, the uptake of health services, breastfeeding duration and women's views of the care they received. Economic evaluation of the implementation of support workers will also be undertaken. The results of the trial should be available at the end of 1999.

■ Conclusion

The quote on the opening page of this chapter portrayed a very bleak picture of the organisation and 'dissipated' focus of postnatal care. It is to be hoped that the results of the trials in progress and the renewed interest of health professionals in the outcome of the whole 'maternity episode', rather than just the pregnancy and the birth, will lead to the provision of postnatal care organised to meet each woman's individual needs.

■ Recommendations for clinical practice in the light of currently available evidence

The results of trials currently in progress will provide much-needed evidence relating to some aspects of postnatal care. Alterations to the current organisation of postnatal care should not be implemented until results are available and evaluated. The following recommendations can, however, be made based on currently available evidence:

1. The length of stay on the postnatal ward in hospital should be flexible. Some women will prefer early discharge, but this will not suit others. Each woman's particular circumstances should be taken into account.

2. Midwives need to consider carefully the basis for planning selective postnatal visits. Visits should ideally be planned according to each woman's need.

3. Women do not volunteer health problems spontaneously, which means that health professionals need to ask about these as part of their ongoing postnatal care.

■ Practice check

● Are women on your maternity unit's postnatal wards offered a choice about when they would prefer to be discharged home?

● Do you perform routine observations and examinations on postnatal women or do you only perform these according to each woman's individual need?

● Do you really 'selectively' visit women in the postnatal period? If so, on what basis do you plan your visits, and do you ask each woman for her opinion of what she wants from your postnatal care?

● If you are working in the community, do you know what postnatal care the GPs in your locality provide?

● Are you familiar with the findings of studies of postpartum morbidity?

● Do you always liaise with the health visitor regarding any health problems that a woman may have experienced when you discharge her from your care?

■ References

Abbott H, Bick DE, MacArthur C (1997) Health after birth. In Henderson C, Jones K (eds) Essential Midwifery. CV Mosby, London, pp. 285–318.
Alexander J, Garcia J, Marchant S (1997) The BLiPP Study. Final Report. University of Portsmouth/National Perinatal Epidemiology Unit, Oxford.
Allen I, Bourke Dowling S, Williams S (1997) A leading role for midwives? Evaluation of midwifery group practice development projects. Policy Studies Institute, London.
Audit Commission (1997) First class delivery: improving maternity services in England and Wales. Audit Commission, London.
Ball JA (1994) Reactions to Motherhood. The Role of Postnatal Care, 2nd edn. Books for Midwives Press, Hale.
Bick DE, MacArthur C (1995a) Attendance, content and relevance of the six week postnatal examination. Midwifery, 11: 69–73.

Bick DE, MacArthur C (1995b) The extent, severity and effect of health problems after childbirth. British Journal of Midwifery 3(1): 27–31.

Bick D, MacArthur C, Winter H *et al* (1997) Redesigning postnatal care: physical and psychological needs. British Journal of Midwifery, 5(10): 621–2.

Bick D, MacArthur C, Fortune H, Winter H (1998) Hospital postnatal care. British Journal of Midwifery, 6(3): 194 (letter).

Bowers J (1985) Is the six–week postnatal examination necessary? Practitioner, 229: 1113–15.

Campbell R, Macfarlane A (1994) Where To Be Born? The Debate and the Evidence, 2nd edn. National Perinatal Epidemiology Unit, Oxford.

Central Midwives Board (1983) Notice Concerning a Midwife's Code of Practice. Central Midwives Board, London.

Cox JL, Holden JM, Sagovsky R (1987) Detection of postnatal depression: development of the Edinburgh postnatal depression scale. British Journal of Psychiatry, 150: 782–6.

Department of Health (1993) Changing Childbirth. The Report of the Expert Maternity Group. HMSO, London.

Dowswell T, Piercy J, Hirst J, Hewison T, Lilford R (1997) For debate. Short postnatal hospital stay: implications for women and service providers. Journal of Public Health Medicine, 19(2): 132–6.

Fillmore M, Miedema G (1996) Cradle. A service offering natural home maternity care. Midwives, 109(1296): 18–19.

Foster K, Lader D, Cheesbrough S (1997) Infant Feeding 1995. Stationery Office, London.

Garcia J, Marchant S (1993) Back to normal? Postpartum health and illness. In Robinson S, Thomson A, Tickner V (eds) Research and the Midwife. Conference Proceedings 1992, University of Manchester, pp. 2–9.

Garcia J, Renfrew M, Marchant S (1994) Postnatal home visiting by midwives. Midwifery, 10: 40–43.

Garcia J, Campbell R, Sandall J, Stevens T, MacKeith N (1997) Assessing the impact on care givers of changes in care. In Campbell R, Garcia J (eds) The Organization of Maternity Care. A Guide to Evaluation. Hochland & Hochland, Hale, pp. 65–78.

Garcia J, Redshaw M, Fitzsimmons B, Keene J (1998) First Class Delivery. A National Survey of Women's Views of Maternity Care. Audit Commission, London.

Glazener CMA (1997) Sexual function after childbirth: women's experiences, persistent morbidity and lack of professional recognition. British Journal of Obstetrics and Gynaecology, 104: 330–5.

Glazener CMA, Abdalla M, Stroud P, Naji S, Templeton A, Russell IT (1995) Postnatal maternal morbidity: extent, causes, prevention and treatment. British Journal of Obstetrics and Gynaecology, 102: 282–7.

Hamilton M (1998) Patterns of postnatal visiting: the views of women and midwives. British Journal of Midwifery, 6(1): 15–18.

House of Commons Health Committee (1992) Second Report. Maternity Services, vol. 1. HMSO, London.

Kroll D, Dwyer D (1994) Postnatal care: teamwork in the community. Modern Midwife (Oct) 10–13.

Kumar R, Robson KM (1984) A prospective study of emotional disorders in childbearing women. British Journal of Psychiatry, 144: 35–47.

Leap N, Hunter B (1993) The Midwife's Tale: An Oral History from Handywoman to Professional Midwife. Scarlett Press, London.

MacArthur C, Lewis M, Knox EG (1991) Health After Childbirth. HMSO, London.

McCourt C, Page L (1996) Report on the evaluation of one-to-one midwifery. Thames Valley University/Hammersmith Hospitals NHS Trust.

Marchant S, Garcia J (1995) Routine clinical care in the immediate postnatal period. In Alexander J, Levy V, Roch S (eds) Aspects of Midwifery Practice. A Research-Based Approach. Macmillan, Basingstoke, pp. 77–91.

Marchant S, Garcia J, Alexander J, Kirkham M (1998) Hospital postnatal care. British Journal of Midwifery, 6(3): 194 (letter).

Marsh J and Sargent E (1991) Factors affecting the duration of postnatal visits. Midwifery, 7: 177–82.

Morrell CJ, Spiby H, Crowther S (1997) Postnatal social support: counting the cost. British Journal of Midwifery, 5(10): 613–15.

RCM Scottish Board/Scottish Health Visitors Association (1995) Partners in Practice. An Exploration of Collaborative Working in Maternity Care Between Health Visitors and Midwives for the Benefit of Mothers, Babies and Families. RCM Scottish Board, Edinburgh.

Renfrew MJ, Lang S (1998) Early vs late discharge postpartum (Cochrane Review) In Cochrane Library, Issue 2, 1998. Oxford: Update Software.

Rider A (1984) Management – A manager's approach to the organisation of normal postnatal care. Midwives Chronicle and Nursing Notes, (Oct suppl.): ii–iv.

Saadeh R, Akre J (1996) Ten steps to successful breastfeeding: a summary of the rationale and scientific evidence. Birth, 23(3): 154–60.

Sharif K, Clarke P, Whittle M (1993) Routine six weeks postnatal examination: to do or not to do? Journal of Obstetrics and Gynaecology, 4(13): 251–2.

Towler J, Bramall J (1986) Midwives in History and Society. Croom Helm, Beckenham.

Twaddle S, Liao X, Fyvie H (1993) An evaluation of postnatal care individualised to the needs of the woman. Midwifery, 9: 154–60.

United Kingdom Central Council for Nursing, Midwifery and Health Visiting (1986) Midwife's Code of Practice. UKCC, London.

United Kingdom Central Council for Nursing, Midwifery and Health Visiting (1993) Midwives' Rules. UKCC, London.

Walsh D (1997) Hospital postnatal care: the end is nigh. British Journal of Midwifery, 5(9): 516–18.

Woolridge MW (1996) Problems of establishing lactation. Food and Nutrition Bulletin, 17(4): 316–23.

■ Suggested Further Reading

Allen I, Bourke Dowling S, Williams S (1997) A Leading Role for Midwives? Evaluation of Midwifery Group Practice Development Projects. Policy Studies Institute, London.

Ball JA (1994) Reactions to Motherhood. The Role of Postnatal Care, 2nd edn. Books for Midwives Press, Hale, Cheshire.

Campbell R, Garcia J (eds) (1997) The Organization of Maternity Care. A Guide to Evaluation. Hochland and Hochland, Hale, Cheshire.

Index